THE HOME REFERENCE TO

HOLISTIC HEALTH

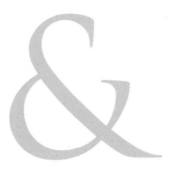

HEALING

THE HOME REFERENCE TO

HOLISTIC HEALTH

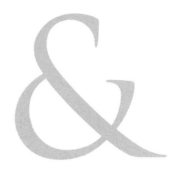

HEALING

Easy-to-Use Natural
Remedies, Herbs, Flower
Essences, Essential
Oils, Supplements, and
Therapeutic Practices for
Health, Happiness, and
Well-Being

Brigitte Mars and Chrystle Fiedler,
Authors of *The Country Almanac of Home Remedies*

Fair Winds Press
100 Cummings Center, Suite 406L
Beverly, MA 01915

fairwindspress.com • bodymindbeautyhealth.com

© 2015 Fair Winds Press

First published in the USA in 2015 by
Fair Winds Press, a member of
Quarto Publishing Group USA Inc.
100 Cummings Center
Suite 406-L
Beverly, MA 01915-6101
www.fairwindspress.com
Visit www.bodymindbeautyhealth.com. It's your personal guide to a happy,
healthy, and extraordinary life!

19 18 17 16 15   1 2 3 4 5

ISBN: 978-1-59233-636-4

Digital edition published in 2015
eISBN: 978-1-62788-180-7

Library of Congress Cataloging-in-Publication Data available

Book design by Claire MacMaster | barefoot art graphic design
All illustrations by Dayna Safferstein Illustration

Printed and bound in China

*The information in this book is for educational purposes only. It is not
intended to replace the advice of a physician or medical practitioner.
Please see your health care provider before beginning any new health program.*

From Brigitte:

*This book is dedicated to my three amazing grandchildren,
Jade Destiny, Solwyn Forest, and Luna Zara.*

From Chrystle:

For Joann Elizabeth Tamin (JET), lover and protector of Mother Earth.

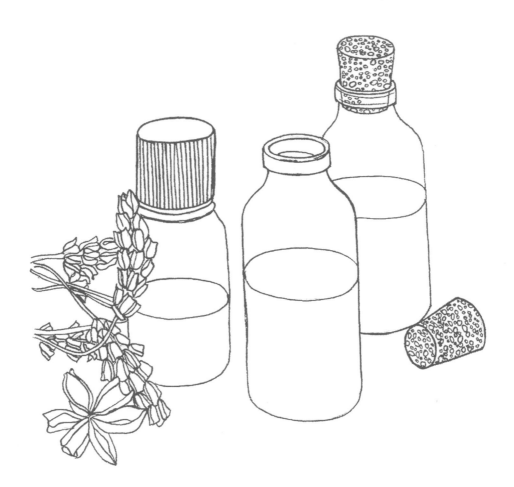

Contents

Foreword

I AM ALWAYS MOVED BY THE GRACE, wisdom, *joie de vivre*, and charismatic charm that Brigitte Mars brings to life and shares so generously with others through her teachings, books, and classes. The numerous books she's written on herbs and natural health are among my favorite herbal references and are frequently on my recommended reading lists for students. They are also on the rather hefty shelf of go-to books I refer too most often when seeking reliable herbal information. Brigitte writes not only from her years of experience as an herbal practitioner, but also weaves together a wide spectrum of natural healing modalities she's integrated into her practice. Her books are always comprehensive, well-researched, user-friendly, and practical.

Chrystle, too, has had a long love affair with herbs and natural remedies and has combined her interest in alternative medicine with her excellent communication and writing skills. She's authored several excellent books on natural healing, including *Beat Sugar Addiction Now!* and *The Complete Idiots Guide to Natural Remedies*, and has written numerous articles on natural health for major publications. Her latest offerings are a fictional mystery series that feature natural remedies. Together, she and Brigitte teamed up to co-author *The Country Almanac of Home Remedies*.

So when I was asked to write the foreword for their most recent book, I was delighted and honored. Though I was expecting it to be, at least, as interesting and comprehensive as the other books they've written, I was even more deeply impressed. *The Home Reference to Holistic Health and Healing* is quite simply one of the best self-help books available on natural therapies for mental and emotional well-being. It contains a wealth of information, tools, and insightful suggestions to help one deal with the daily stresses of modern life as well the illnesses and imbalances that arise from an overly stressed system.

It is estimated that more than 100 million Americans suffer from stress-related problems and that stress-related issues account for more than 80 percent of visits to the doctor. Yet many of these issues and visits can be circumvented by understanding the underlying problem(s) and are often resolved by natural remedies and lifestyle changes. Although there are undoubtedly times when medical intervention is necessary and lifesaving—and this book clearly points to that direction when needed—most of the daily stress-related issues we encounter are safely and effectively treated by less invasive and equally effective home remedies.

Mental and emotional well-being are essential for health and are as equally important as physical health, yet are often overlooked. Our go-go culture doesn't allow time for nurturing the soul, but it's essential for a happy, joyful life. The healing power of herbs and other natural practices can help do just that. Natural cures help soothe stress, ease anxiety, and boost mood, immunity, mental acuity, and energy, and make room in our lives for joy and happiness. This book is filled with the best suggestions for just how to do that, and equally important, gives practical step-by-step instructions.

Although Americans are just waking up to the power of herbal and natural medicine, these practices are as old as civilization itself. According to the World Health Organization, 80 percent of the world uses herbal and natural remedies as a primary source of health care. The Natural Pharmacy reports that one out of every three adult Americans uses complementary and alternative medical care.

There is no denying that conventional (allopathic) medicine is making amazing progress today, and is an essential path of treatment if you have severe mental and emotional challenges. Any life-threatening illness needs to be treated by a competent health professional.

Alternatively, herbs, whether in capsule, tincture, salve, or tea, are the medicine of the home, helping us to be more self-reliant and proactive in our own health. Herbs are most effectively used for non-emergency health problems that pop up in daily life. Problems such as stress, anxiety, mild depression, low energy and immunity, and sleep and memory issues are among the many imbalances that can be effectively, safely, and inexpensively treated at home.

Rather than curing illnesses, plants and herbal medicine are best at preventing them. By providing rich nutrients that can help to bolster the body's immunity, we can often mobilize the immune system and, in turn, its ability to fight off infections before we get sick. When we eat medicinal plants or use them in some way, we become hardier, more tenacious and disease-resistant, just as our favorite weeds are in the wild—and in our gardens!

Holistic healing works in myriad ways. For example, learning how to naturally manage stress, the root of a majority of modern illnesses, will help you not only feel better today but may also help prevent it from manifesting into a serious illness, such as heart disease or stroke, down the line. Herbal and natural cures create a foundation of wellness by addressing the root of chronic health problems, which can include lifestyle choices, environmental factors, and genetics. *The Home Reference to Holistic*

Health and Healing is full of lifestyle and dietary suggestions along with herbal remedies, and natural and holistic therapies that can address these problems and begin the healing process.

Herbal medicine and other time-tested holistic practices can help you find lasting solutions for mental health and healing and can make you healthier than you've ever been before, in mind, body, and spirit. The good news is that these cures can be used in conjunction with conventional medicine under the guidance of a doctor. The choice is up to you.

Brigitte and Chrystle are long-time soul sisters when it comes to herbal and holistic medicine. So, I have no doubt that you'll benefit from their wise, health-giving, joyful advice. Like each of their other books, *The Home Reference to Holistic Health and Healing* is written in that eminently practical and self-empowering manner that's a signature of their work. Read, practice, enjoy, and be at peace.

In Joy,
Rosemary Gladstar
Herbalist & Author
From her home on Sage Mountain, Vermont

GREETINGS! Get ready to learn hundreds of natural ways to improve the many functions of your brain, nervous system, and emotional health so that you can be your brightest self for the highest good.

So many people suffer from common concerns such as stress, depression, anxiety, pain, and others that can drain the possibilities of a joyful life. We grow through the hardships in life, but they can be incapacitating when we have a job to do, children to raise, and all the rigors of life before us.

Simply relying on medication to get us through trying times can take its own toll, leading to physical side effects, low energy, diminished libido, weight gain, and even organ damage.

What You'll Find Here

The Home Reference to Holistic Health and Healing offers time-tested, natural methods to help you manage life's mental and emotional challenges. It addresses lifestyle techniques, food choices, herbal remedies, essential oils, vitamin supplements, homeopathy, and flower essences that can help nourish and support your body and mind so that each challenge becomes an opportunity to grow stronger than ever.

A Brief History of Natural Cures for Health

Methods for treating mental disorders have varied through the ages. Asclepius (considered one of the fathers of medicine, about 130 BCE) restored balance with massage, fresh air, diet, and exercise. He was one of the first to release insane people from the confinements of dark cellars and recommended occupational therapy, calming herbs, soothing music, and exercise to improve attention and memory.

Hippocrates placed the site of mental functioning in the brain and speculated that those with mental illness were imbalanced in the humours: bile, wind, and phlegm. He introduced the terms *melancholy* and *mania*.

During the Middle Ages, there was belief in supernatural causes of mental disease, including evil spirits, the stars, and wicked spells. During the Renaissance, the emphasis again shifted toward more natural causes of mental illness, though there was little change in the actual treatment of it.

Historically, depression (and insanity) was treated by whipping, bloodletting, exorcism, and water treatments (cold plunges, showers, and sprays). Thankfully, kindness has mostly replaced brutality.

Before We Start, a Few Caveats

I promise you no torture here, but please heed a few cautions:

- If you use prescription drugs, avoid mixing them with alcohol.
- Never use someone else's prescriptions to treat your symptoms, and don't use more than the prescribed dosage.
- Make sure your health care professional is aware of any other substances you are taking, including herbs, vitamins, and other drugs.
- If you're on medication, stay on it unless otherwise instructed by your doctor.
- Talk to a competent health professional about any contraindications with foods, drugs, herbs, or vitamins.

The Value of Holistic Care

Remember that specialists filter your ailments through their expertise. Your chiropractor might believe your headaches are due to pinched nerves, while a neurologist might want to consider a brain tumor. In truth, you might just need to cut back on coffee. This is why holistic physicians and other health care providers can be invaluable, as they look at the whole you rather than you as the sum of your parts.

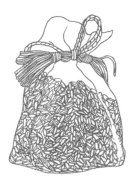

Make Changes
to Your Life Slowly

When you decide to rely more on the power of natural remedies for mental and emotional health, it's important to talk to your health professional about gradually decreasing pharmaceuticals in a safe way. One suggestion is to reduce a drug dosage by one-eighth every two to four weeks. It is best to avoid mixing drugs and herbs within three hours of each other.

While detoxing from drugs, taking a vitamin C and B complex supplement can aid in detoxification. Choose the strategy that suits you and adjust as needed.

Most importantly, listen to your own wisdom about your body. Tune in to your cycles. Instead of rushing through your day and life, slow down and allow yourself to find your true rhythm.

Take this guided journey to learn simple, natural, healthy ways to encourage and improve a healthy mind, psyche, and emotional being, all of which are affected by the healthy (or unhealthy) ways we treat our body.

Explore and learn how to use simple, time-tested techniques to feel and heal. Thank you for this opportunity to be a guide on the path of your well-being.

Peace & blessings,

Brigitte Mars, A.H.G.

Introduction

THE FIRST BOOK IN THIS SERIES, *The Country Almanac of Home Remedies,* focused on natural cures for all types of common conditions and ailments. In *The Home Reference to Holistic Health and Healing,* you'll learn how to take the next step, using natural remedies to improve your overall health, happiness, and well-being.

Natural cures can help you tackle big life challenges, such as reducing stress, anxiety, and depression; maximizing sleep; managing chronic pain; and gaining mental acuity for a more balanced and joyful life.

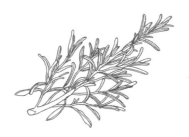

Why Use Natural Remedies?

More people than ever before are turning to natural remedies. According to the National Center for Complementary and Alternative Medicine (NCCAM), more than 42 percent of Americans use integrative medicine, which combines alternative and conventional medicine. It's no surprise. As opposed to conventional cures, natural remedies work *with* the body's own innate processes to speed healing instead of suppressing symptoms with medications.

The Latest Research into Natural Remedies

Numerous medical studies prove the efficacy of natural cures for improving health, happiness, and well-being. In 2004, NCCAM began to fund research studies on herbal medicine. This has added to the already burgeoning wealth of knowledge we have about natural medicines, first as folk remedies, now as mainstream medicine. Many studies showing the efficacy of natural cures have come out of Europe, specifically Germany: In 1978, West Germany appointed a panel of experts, called Commission E, to study herbs to treat different health conditions.

Why Do You Need This Book?

Considering the economy, world politics and conflicts, and day-to-day living, more people are stressed out than ever before. Estimates are that more than 100 million Americans suffer from a stress-related problem. Although studies show that a little stress can be beneficial, prolonged stress is not and can result in the following conditions:

- Chronic illness
- Depression
- Higher risk of stroke and heart attack
- Impaired immune function
- Accidents
- Cancer
- Lung disease

It is estimated that 80 percent of doctor visits are due to stress-related illnesses. Natural remedies such as herbs (think chamomile tea for stress and anxiety); vitamins, minerals, and food-based nutrients (fish oil for better moods and brain power); supplements; flower essences (rosemary essential oil for memory); and therapeutic practices such as yoga, aromatherapy, meditation, relaxation response, homeopathy, acupuncture, massage, walking, and even gardening can ease the symptoms of stress-related conditions and improve overall health and well-being.

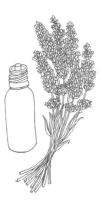

Natural Remedies Are Safe

Natural cures generally have fewer side effects because they're not as concentrated as prescription drugs, which are synthesized with chemicals to make them strong. Most natural remedies are safe when used as directed because they are designed to work with the body. This is good news for people who are also worried about overdosing and addiction.

Saving Money with Natural Remedies

Natural remedies are typically a less expensive way to improve one's well-being. Natural remedies also support a healthier planet. What would you rather have in your neighborhood? A field of lavender or a smokestack spewing toxic fumes into the air and water?

How to Use This Book

Think of *The Home Reference to Holistic Health and Healing* as your new mind-body-spirit reference book. Here you'll find solutions from time-tested natural remedies proven by the latest research. In each chapter you'll find specific advice and information that you can use right now to feel better and enjoy life more.

You'll also find an overview of each condition or aspect of happiness. Next, you'll learn about the types of natural remedies that can help to restore balance and make you feel better. The natural remedies are in these categories:

 Necessary Nutrients: Feeding the brain and the central nervous system with the right foods

 Well-Being Supplements: Vitamins and minerals that can help

 Healing Herbs: For health and well-being

Natural Practices: Meditation, yoga, exercise, gardening, breath work, homeopathy, aromatherapy, and flower essences

 Holistic Therapies: Massage, acupuncture, and acupressure (with DIY instructions)

Sidebars such as Mother Nature's News (timely studies that show the effectiveness of natural cures), Thrifty Cures (remedies that cost very little), Skip This! (practices to avoid), Good to Grow! (remedies you can grow yourself), Good to Know! (surprising or important information), Cure Caution (warnings or precautions), and When to See Your M.D. supplement the text and will guide you on your journey to health and well-being.

You will also find a treasure trove of information in the appendices. Learn in-depth about everything from homeopathy to aromatherapy to color therapy and put it to use in your life.

But before you get started, please read the section below on safety and refer to it as needed.

Safety First

Before using any of the herbs listed in this book first check the essential herbs in appendix A for any contraindications, such as what to avoid during pregnancy, when nursing, or when taking prescription drugs. Mixing herbs with prescription drugs can cause exacerbated or unpredictable effects. This is especially the case when you are using an herb for the same purpose as a drug. You may end up with a double dose.

Remember: If you're taking prescription medication, don't take any herbs that are not regarded as safe for all persons without first checking with your health care practitioner.

If you're taking medication for a particular ailment, you shouldn't also take herbs for that ailment without first checking with your health care practitioner.

It may be wise to gradually decrease the amount of drugs while gradually increasing the amount of herbs taken internally over a period of time rather than making any abrupt changes, while improving diet and lifestyle. Talk to your health practitioner for guidance.

Separating drugs from herbs for at least three hours is also a beneficial practice, as many combinations have not been tried or tested.

Dosage Guidelines

Dosages will depend in part on the herbs you're thinking about using. If you're using a commercial product, always follow the dosage guidelines on the product packaging.

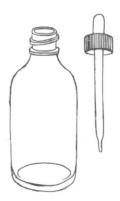

If you've made your own tea or tincture, in general, one 8-ounce cup (235 ml) of tea or one dropperful of tincture qualifies as a single dose. For an acute, serious, right-there-in-your-face type of illness, one dose every hour or two would be appropriate except while sleeping—rest is good medicine in its own right.

For a chronic health concern, one dose three or four times daily would be appropriate. Some herbalists recommend pulsing remedies for chronic conditions, which means ten days on, three days off, in a continuing cycle. Pulsing helps the body acclimate and learn to respond even without the herbs. Another pulsing regimen is six days on, one day off, with a three-day break every two or three weeks.

When you are using herbs for therapeutic purposes, continue with the appropriate dosage for at least a week and then evaluate your progress. If your health concern has been remedied, you can stop taking the herb formula on a regular basis. However, you might wish to include some of it in your diet from time to time as a tonic tune-up.

Special Situations

The dosage guidelines discussed above are generally effective for adults. However, dosages may need to be adjusted for different people or different categories of people. For example:

- Large people may need a higher dose than small people.
- Women may need less than men.
- For dosages for the elderly, reduce the dose by one-fourth for those over sixty-five and by one-half for those over seventy.

For Herbs

In general, one cup of tea equals one dropperful of tincture, which equals two capsules or tablets. If dealing with an acute condition, such as an infection, it may be necessary to use either one cup of tea, a dropperful of tincture, or two capsules or tablets every two waking hours, at least for a couple of days. Then, as the condition improves, space those dosages further apart.

Avoid Interactions

Usually four pellets are placed under the tongue and allowed to dissolve. It is best to not eat or drink anything for ten minutes before or after taking the remedy to avoid interfering with its effectiveness. Some homeopaths recommend avoiding coffee, mint, and camphor while using homeopathic remedies.

For Vitamins

Check the label for dosage suggestions.

For Essential Oils

Do not use essential oils internally unless properly trained. For external use, use two drops of pure essential oil to 1 tablespoon (15 ml) of carrier oil such as grapeseed oil. Lavender and tea tree oil can be applied undiluted (neat), using no more than five drops at a time. Avoid using essential oils topically during pregnancy.

If you have any questions, please consult your health care practitioner for guidance. This is especially true with conditions such as depression, which may need careful supervision.

Chapter 1

NATURE'S REMEDIES, THERAPIES, AND PRACTICES FROM A–Z

The greatest affliction of the cosmos is never to have been afflicted. Mortals only learn wisdom by experiencing tribulation.
—The Urantia Book

According to the *Journal of the American Medical Association*, people turn to alternative healing because of its focus on the mind–body connection and the fact that remedies can be tailored to each person's individual needs. In this chapter, you'll learn about the wide variety of natural remedies, therapies, and practices, from aromatherapy and acupuncture to flower essences, herbs, and homeopathy—and their many benefits.

Acupuncture

An estimated 8.2 million U.S. adults have used acupuncture, a practice from Traditional Chinese Medicine (TCM). TCM is based on the belief that disease results when chi, or the vital life force in the body, is disrupted and an imbalance of yin and yang occurs. Yin represents the cold, slow, or passive principle, while yang represents the hot, excited, or active principle.

There are twelve main meridians, eight secondary meridians, and more than two thousand acupuncture points on the human body that connect with them. Acupuncture stimulates these points on the body when thin metal needles are inserted into the skin to relieve blockages to chi and improve health. Acupressure, a similar concept, uses fingertips to stimulate the body's acupoints.

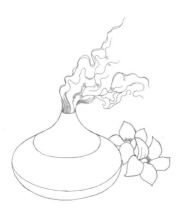

Acupuncture's benefits may come from releasing pain-killing neurochemicals, such as endorphins and immune system cells, at specific sites in the body. Studies show that acupuncture can help reduce or improve headache, menstrual cramps, tennis elbow, fibromyalgia, osteoarthritis of the knee, lower back pain, carpal tunnel syndrome, and asthma.

Aromatherapy

Aromatherapy is the practice of using essential plant oils to heal the body, mind, and spirit. One of the most ancient methods of aromatherapy was to burn aromatic branches and inhale the smoke. The word *perfume* is derived from the Latin *per fumum*, meaning "through smoke."

Essential oils, also known as volatile oils, are distilled or pressed from plants and flowers. In nature, essential oils help protect plants from fungi, bacteria, and viruses. They help repel predator insects and attract beneficial pollinators.

In humans, the fragrance of essential oil reaches the nose, travels along a neurological pathway, bypassing the blood–brain barrier, and eventually enters the bloodstream, where it stimulates neurotransmitter production and affects your moods. Essential oils are also believed to interrupt the oxygenation cycles of bacteria as well as interact with the receptor sites in the central nervous system.

Genuine aromatherapy utilizes only essential oils derived directly from plants. Be sure you use pure essential plant oils and not synthetic fragrances. Keep essential oils away from infants, toddlers, and children. For more information on aromatherapy and the "essential oil medicine cabinet," see Appendix B.

Craniosacral Therapy

Craniosacral therapy was developed in the 1970s by osteopathic physician and surgeon John E. Upledger, D.O., O.M.M. This therapy helps release restrictions in the membranes around the brain and spinal cord so the central nervous system can perform more effectively.

For this therapy you lie down on a massage or treatment table. Using a very light touch (about the weight of a nickel), the practitioner tests for restrictions in the craniosacral system by monitoring the rhythm of the cerebrospinal fluid and releases any blockages to help the body heal and restore balance.

Flower Essences

Bach Flower Essences were discovered by noted homeopath and bacteriologist Edward Bach, M.D., in England more than seventy-five years ago. Flower essences are made from a "sun tea" of specific wildflowers or trees known for their healing properties, then diluted (similar to homeopathic remedies) and used to balance emotions and encourage healing. Bach Flower Remedies are dispensed over the counter and have no contraindications or side effects. They're nontoxic, nonaddictive, and safe, even for infants, the elderly, plants, and animals. Visit www.bachcentre.com for a complete list of Bach Foundation Registered Practitioners.

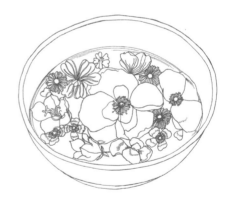

Bach Original Flower Remedies and What They Treat

Agrimony: You hide your troubles behind a smile.

Aspen: You are anxious but can't say why.

Beech: You feel intolerant toward others.

Centaury: You can't easily say no to others.

Cerato: You know what you want to do but doubt your judgment.

Cherry plum: You feel that you might lose mental control.

Chestnut bud: You find yourself making the same mistakes.

Chicory: Your possessive love for your family makes it hard to let go.

Clematis: You are in a dream.

Crab apple: You feel unclean and/or dislike something about yourself.

Elm: You feel overwhelmed by your many responsibilities.

Gentian: You feel a bit let down after a setback.

Gorse: You give up when things go wrong.

Heather: Your self-centeredness leads to loneliness.

Holly: You feel wounded, jealous, spiteful, or vengeful.

Honeysuckle: Your mind is on the past rather than the present.

Hornbeam: You put things off, feeling tired at the thought of starting work.

Impatiens: You feel impatient with the slow pace of people or things.

Larch: You expect to fail and lack confidence in your skills.

Mimulus: You feel shy or anxious about something specific.

Mustard: You feel down in the dumps and don't know why.

Oak: You go beyond the limits of your strength.

Olive: You feel tired after making an effort.

Pine: You feel guilty or blame yourself.

Red chestnut: You feel anxious about somebody else's safety.

Rock rose: You are terrified about something.

Rock water: You are rigid in your outlook and practice self-denial.

Scleranthus: You can't make your mind up.

Star of Bethlehem: You are suffering from the effects of shock or grief.

Sweet chestnut: You feel despair when there is no hope left.

Vervain: Your enthusiasm leads you to burn yourself out.

Vine: Sometimes you are a tyrant when you want to lead.

Walnut: Other people's ideas knock you off course, or you are unsettled at times of change.

Water violet: You like your own company but sometimes feel lonely.

White chestnut: Your mind is running over the same thing.

Wild oat: You want to do something worthwhile but can't find your vocation, or you have uncertainty in your direction in life.

Wild rose: You can't really be bothered.

Willow: You feel both resentful and sorry for yourself.

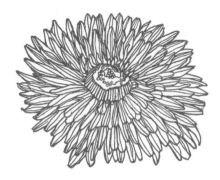

Herbal Remedies

To this day, between 25 and 30 percent of modern drugs have their basis in plant medicine. Nations send ethnobotanists and pharmacognosists into remote portions of the globe to observe what more "primitive" peoples are using in healing. When the plants are brought home, the quest begins for the "active ingredient," which is very often an alkaloid. Some examples of alkaloids include caffeine, morphine, nicotine, cocaine, quinine, and salacin, many of which are made into strong drugs. Yet a plant is not solely an alkaloid. Botanicals contain a powerhouse of plant intelligence, including chlorophyll, essential oils, glycosides, vitamins, minerals, and other secondary components—many of which increase the plants' effectiveness and help to prevent side effects. Herbs have been time-tested for thousands of years by millions of people.

Homeopathy

Homeopathy is based on the law of similars, or the philosophy that "like cures like." The term *homeopathy* comes from the Greek words *homeo*, meaning "similar," and *pathos*, meaning "suffering or disease," and was developed by German physician Samuel Hahnemann (1755–1843). Each solution contains an infinitesimal amount of the substance; you might say it contains a pattern replica of the substance. Exposure to the pattern replica, however, triggers a powerful healing response from the body. In other words, by stimulating the body's own healing response, a homeopathic remedy encourages the body to heal itself.

Homeopathic remedies can effect amazingly fast-acting and profound cures. The degree of success, however, depends on selecting the right remedy for a person's constitution, so although you can diagnose and treat yourself, you may also benefit from consultation with a professional homeopath to gain insight into the best remedies for your constitution. Note that homeopathy often calls for very small doses of substances that in large doses could be toxic. *Do not confuse homeopathic remedies with herbal remedies.*

Homeopathic remedies come in the form of small pellets, alcohol solutions, and water solutions and are usually safe when taken with conventional drugs. Contact your health practitioner if your symptoms do not improve within five days or if you are pregnant or nursing. Keep the remedy out of the reach of children. You'll find out more information about homeopathic remedies on page 31.

Massage Therapy

Massage therapy is performed by using long, smooth strokes and kneading soft tissue and muscles, improving circulation, fostering detoxification and lymph drainage, and enhancing immune function. Because many illnesses are stress related, massage improves health by helping you to relax. According to the American Massage Therapy Association, 71 percent of hospitals and clinics offer massage therapy for stress management. Different types of therapy include Swedish massage (most common), aromatherapy massage (with essential oils), hot stone massage (using heated, smooth stones), deep tissue massage (targets deeper levels of muscles and connective tissue), and Shiatsu (a type of Japanese bodywork). The act of being touched is also good for mind, body, and spirit.

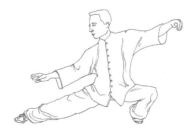

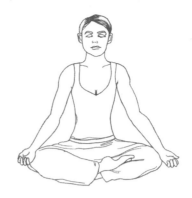

Meditation

Millions of people around the planet regularly meditate, a mind-body practice that uses certain techniques such as focused attention (on a word, an object, or the breath, for example), a specific posture, and a neutral attitude toward distracting thoughts and emotions. Over time, meditation enables you to quiet what is called the "monkey mind," the thinking that just won't stop, and rest in peaceful awareness of your true self.

Qigong

Qigong (*Qi* [chi] means "energy" and *gong* [kung] means "a skill or a practice") originated 5,000 years ago when Chinese scholars studying the workings of the universe concluded that everything is energy, as did Albert Einstein much later. The theory of qigong is that you become sick when energy in the body is out of balance, too much, or not enough. Qigong practice helps to change the flow of energy in the body, resulting in improved wellness.

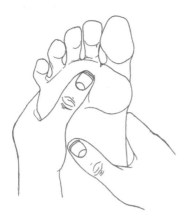

Reflexology

Reflexology dates back to ancient Egypt, India, and China and is the practice of stimulating nerves in the feet, hands, and ears to improve health. Practitioners work on pressure points that correspond to areas of the body. Reflexology assists the self-healing process by balancing life energy, or qi, in the body. So, for example, when you rub the point between your index finger and your thumb (L4, or large intestine 4), you treat the pain of migraine headaches.

Yoga

Sixteen-and-a-half million Americans now practice yoga, a 5,000-year-old spiritual practice that began in India. By performing poses (asanas), you find health and vitality through increased oxygen intake and the release of feel-good endorphins. Yoga also improves flexibility, strength, and muscle tone and reduces stress.

There are many different types of yoga, including hatha and Kripalu yoga. Yoga nidra or what is known as "yogic sleep" is gaining popularity and is easy to do. You just need to lie down and rest in savasana or corpse pose while a teacher (or CD) instructs you in a guided meditation/visualization through the five koshas, or states of mind and body, including the body, breath, and emotions. This practice helps remove emotional barriers and judgments so you can relax into self-acceptance.

The practice works by triggering the relaxation response in your parasympathetic nervous system—an antidote to the fight-or-flight instinct that revs us up in stressful situations. The practice also engages the hippocampus and the frontal cortex of the brain, which improves clarity and moderates the amygdala, which helps create calm and replace negative patterns with more positive ones.

Chapter 2

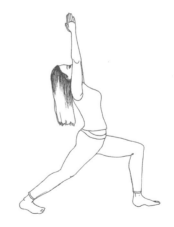

TAME STRESS

There is more to life than increasing its speed.
—Mohandas K. Gandhi

Learning how to manage stress and stressful situations is one of the most important tasks on your journey to a happier life. Stress is caused by anything that disturbs our serenity and makes us feel unsafe. From the economy, technology, politics, and the state of the world to relationships, child care, money, living situations, or sudden or chronic illness, large and small changes alike (even positive ones) cause stress. Most of us think of stress as a nuisance, but we rarely examine the cost it has on our lives, our health, and the way it causes "dis-ease" in the body.

The Body's Response to Stress

Feeling stressed out activates the fight-or-flight response, which means hormones such as adrenaline and cortisol are released in the body. When this happens, the heart rate increases so that blood is available to supply the muscles, respiratory rate and sweat production accelerate, and blood sugar levels elevate as the liver releases stored glucose into the bloodstream.

Ideally, we would experience stress and relax once the danger was over. But because we have a central cortex, stressful images and the feelings they provoke have a long shelf life, leaving us chronically stressed, impairing immune system function, and causing inflammation in the body, which can lead to chronic diseases such as heart disease, hypertension, and diabetes. Chronic muscle tension makes us more armored because we hold our muscles tightly, which can decrease circulation. It prevents good circulation, impairs digestion, can leave you more prone to illness, and may morph into anxiety.

 Mother Nature's News

Stress Makes You Age Faster

Stress can accelerate the aging process, according to a 2013 study in the medical journal *Proceedings of the National Academy of Sciences*. Researchers at the University of California at San Francisco studied thirty-nine women ages twenty to fifty who were caring for a chronically ill child.

They studied telomeres, the caps at the ends of our chromosomes that become shorter and shrivel when we age, and concluded that chronic stress speeds up this process. The women who were the most stressed had telomeres equal to someone ten years older.

 Good to Know!

It's easy when we're stressed to stop doing good things for ourselves. Instead, think of it as an opportunity to take better care of yourself and focus on self-care. Though stress may be unavoidable, we can come through most ordeals if lifestyle is balanced by good nutrition; exercise; useful natural remedies, practices, and therapies; rest; and spiritual practice.

Self-Care Defuses Stress

The most effective way to deal with stress is to focus on self-care. Taking small actions every day will help you to defuse stress when it arises, enabling you to return to calm more easily. Think of it as depositing serenity into your well-being bank. If you don't make regular deposits, you won't have the peace of mind that you need to counterbalance stressful situations.

So you don't feel overwhelmed about the process, try incorporating one of the healthy changes in this chapter into your regular routine, whether it's taking fifteen minutes each day for yoga or meditation, adding a new nourishing food to your diet, drinking a daily cup of herbal tea, or journaling about how you feel.

Nourish Your Body with Necessary Nutrients

You are what you eat, especially when it comes to handling stress. Eating a whole-food diet that includes organic vegetables, fruits, legumes, nuts, seeds, and oils provides the nutrients, fiber, and phytochemicals you need to improve your defenses against stress.

Choose nutritious foods; small, frequent meals; and **high-protein** and complex carbohydrates, which help to keep the blood sugar on an even keel as well as providing important B vitamins. **Oatmeal** and **yogurt** are two foods that are easy to digest and rich in calming calcium. Other foods that help ease stress include **almonds**, **raisins**, and **sunflower seeds**. **Onions** contain tension-relieving prostaglandins. Give the stressed-out person warm, nourishing foods rather than cold ones.

Skip This!

Foods that will increase the negative effects of stress include alcohol, caffeinated beverages, fruit juices, and sugar.

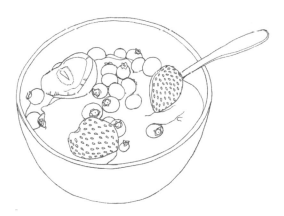

Healing Herbs

Nature's floral pharmacy provides many herbs that nourish and support a frayed nervous system. Taking the time to savor a cup of soothing herbal tea is a wonderful way to nourish your nerves. The act of brewing a cup of tea is also a good way to slow down.

Tasting and enjoying herbal teas also gives you time to reflect on your day and what's next and how best to handle it. As you drink health-giving teas, think healing thoughts, such as "I am enough" and "All is well in my life now." You'll find a lot more detail about making the perfect cup of tea in *The Country Almanac of Home Remedies*.

Calming herbal baths can provide centering and relaxation if you feel stressed. Just put a handful of fresh or dried herbs into a washcloth and close it with a hair tie or rubber band, and throw in into the tub as it is filling. Or use ½ cup of herbs and make a pot of herbal tea, simmer for twenty minutes, and add that to the tub. Use a metal filter when draining to catch any debris, and use it as compost. You can also add eight to ten drops of your favorite essential oil to the bath once it's full. Inhale the aroma and feel yourself relax.

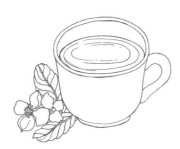

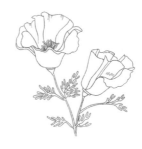

Herbal Stress Relief

These are some herbs that can be used as tea, tincture, or capsules.

Ashwagandha builds chi and helps lower cortisol levels. It makes the body more resistant to stress and prevents depletion of vitamin C.

California poppy is a skeletal relaxant that encourages restoration of the nervous system.

Catnip is a soothing nerve tonic that helps take the edge off.

Chamomile is a gentle relaxant that tones the nervous system.

Eleuthero nourishes the adrenals and is considered an adaptogen that helps people acclimate to stressful situations.

Ginseng helps the body adapt to stress and maintain normal blood pressure, glucose levels, and hormonal function.

Hawthorn calms the spirit and increases circulation to the brain.

Hops contains lupulin, which is considered a strong but safe, reliable sedative.

Kava kava relaxes the muscles without blocking nerve signals and calms physical tension without numbing mental processes.

Lemon balm's volatile oils help protect the cerebrum from excess external stimuli.

Linden calms the nerves and promotes rest.

Oatstraw relaxes the nerves and strengthens the nervous system.

Passionflower quiets the central nervous system and slows the breakdown of neurotransmitters, serotonin, and norepinephrine.

Skullcap calms and strengthens the nerves, relaxes spasms, relieves pain, and promotes rest.

Valerian, a strong central nervous system relaxant, improves poor concentration for those under stress.

Vervain helps strengthen a weakened nervous system.

Wild lettuce calms the nervous system, aids sleep, relaxes the ganglions, and relieves pain.

Wood betony relaxes and strengthens the nerves and relieves pain.

Well-Being Supplements
Stress depletes the body's reserves of vitamins and minerals; using supplements during stressful periods will help you reverse the depletion. Consider a vitamin B complex with C to replenish the water-soluble nutrients. They not only nourish the nervous system but also give you the energy needed to deal with life's problems. Calcium and magnesium (1,000 mg each) help to ease tension and irritability. Our requirements for these nutrients are increased during difficult times.

Good to Know!
One low-tech way to test how your adrenal glands are functioning is to bend over and touch your toes. Dizziness when you return to standing may be a sign of weakened adrenal glands. In what is known as *tongue diagnosis*, a person's tongue may go in and out when he or she is trying to hold it out, and this is another sign of adrenal fatigue.

Banishing Adrenal Burnout
Chronic stress can affect your adrenal glands. The word *adrenal* is Latin for "on the kidneys." In fact, the adrenal glands sit directly on top of the kidneys and produce fluids that enable the kidneys to do their job. Thirty-two known hormones are released from the adrenal glands, including adrenaline. The outer cortex of each adrenal gland secretes corticosteroids, which are made from cholesterol and sex hormones.

Nourishing Nutrients for Adrenal Health
The adrenal glands (as well as the kidneys) benefit from mineral-rich black foods such as black sesame seeds, black rice, black quinoa, and chia seeds. Sunflower seeds are a good tonic food for the adrenal glands. In addition, be sure to get enough protein.

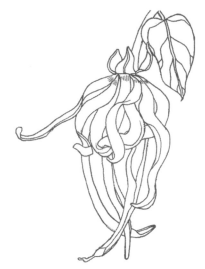

Herbs that are beneficial for strengthening the adrenal glands include:

Astragalus: Enhances the function of the adrenal cortex; can ease exhaustion, incontinence, and weakness.

Burdock root: Aids in the elimination of uric acid.

Eleuthero: Helps the body adapt to a variety of stress factors.

Licorice: Is beneficial for those with Addison's disease and adrenal exhaustion.

Schizandra berries: Is an adaptogen, kidney tonic, rejuvenative, and restorative.

Turmeric: Is an antioxidant.

Aromatherapy Aid for Adrenal Glands

Adrenal-stimulating essential oils to use in aromatherapy include basil, pine, rosemary, and sage. You'll find more information about essential oils in Appendix B.

 Natural Practices

Self-care is one of the most effective ways to defuse stress. Try these natural practices and see.

Aromatherapy

Essential oils that relieve stress include anise, basil, bay leaf, bergamot, cardamom, chamomile, clary sage, cypress, fennel, frankincense, geranium, ginger, helichrysum, jasmine, juniper, lavender, lemon, marjoram, melissa, neroli, nutmeg, orange, peppermint, pine, rose, rosewood, sage, sandalwood, spearmint, tangerine, thyme, and ylang-ylang.

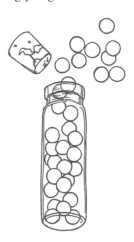

Homeopathy

Homeopathic remedies that can benefit mental and emotional health include:

Aconitum napellus (aconite): Remedy for sudden fright or acute fear. You fear death, darkness, evil, and even crossing the street. Anguish, anxiety, despair, insomnia, restlessness, and franticness are all characteristic of the person who needs aconite. You may panic in crowded places when you fear you cannot get out or fear natural disasters, accidents, and shock or when being reminded of them. You wake up frightened with palpitations. You're sensitive to light, noise, and touch.

Anacardium orientale (cashew): You have anticipatory anxiety, difficulty concentrating, low self-confidence, and fear of failure and insanity.

Argentum nitricum (silver nitrate): You're impulsive and fear impending events, crowds, and heights. You're anxious before an interview or exam. You may have panic attacks and diarrhea when anticipating circumstances.

Arnica (Arnica montana flower): For shock, trauma (physical and emotional), pain, before and after surgery, dentistry, and labor. Usually the first remedy given after a traumatic event. Aids in reabsorption of fibrin, a blood protein that forms as a result of internal injuries, thereby reducing swelling and bruising.

Arsenicum album (white arsenic): You are fussy, obsessive, overanxious, restless, and fearful; you worry about the past and future. Your mind is never at rest, and you toss and turn when sleeping. You want everything to be just right and are always in motion. You're fatigued, fidgety, high-strung, worried, and faultfinding. You fear being alone, losing control, illness, death, and darkness. You usually have a frail constitution and are cold, thin, and always in motion. You may experience vertigo and memory loss.

Aurum metallicum (gold): For lost love, feeling dull and stupid, and happy at the thought of death. Use for depression resulting from personal trauma, when feelings of anger surface and are then suppressed, or business loss, when you feel in deep despair and worthless. Aurum people are often leaders, noble and successful in their fields. When loss or failure occurs, you can feel deeply affected and may turn to prayer. You feel as if a black cloud sits over the future. You feel devalued, sullen, and brooding. You may have been a leader or extremely successful and have substance abuse issues.

Calcarea carbonica (carbonate of lime): You're anxious about health and catching infection. Helps children's fears of the dark, insects, monsters, cats, and dogs. Use for fear of misfortune, disease, insanity, and loss of reason. For tired, anxious people who perspire easily. When you're easily discouraged or methodical. Helps those who break down from overwork.

Calcarea ostrearum (calcium carbonate): You feel sluggish, lazy, and apathetic You have trouble verbalizing, feel old and tired, and often sit around feeling sorry for yourself. You may feel cold, with your feet feeling especially chilled. You may have night sweats, shortness of breath, or feel confused and depressed.

Causticum (lime and potassium bicarbonate): Depression due to death of a parent or friend. You feel negative, gloomy, and anxious. You cry over small things. You feel an anxious foreboding that something is about to happen. May benefit if you cry frequently. You may be experiencing forgetfulness and mental dullness. You worry about others rather than yourself.

Chamomilla (chamomile): For angry children or those constantly discontent. For anxiety and impatience. For when you cry out in sleep.

Coffea cruda (coffee): For paralyzing anxiety preceding an event such as flying or public speaking. Mental activity causes insomnia. You are excited and nervous.

Gelsemium (yellow jasmine): You are paralyzed with grief following a loss and may tremble. You can't cry. For mild depression following an illness such as the flu. For anxiety based on fear, including exams and stage fright. You're trembling and may freeze up physically and mentally.

Hypericum (Saint-John's-wort): For nerve injury to areas with lots of nerves, such as fingers, toes, and spine. Can help prevent the need for stitches. For crushing injuries and sharp, shooting pain. For old injuries with nerves that still hurt. Use after dental work. Often referred to as "arnica for the nerves."

Ignatia (St. Ignatius' bean): Use for disappointment in love or death. For acute loss such as that of a child, parent, friend, or pet. The bereaved person has strongly identified with the person lost and feels they cannot exist without them. Use for grieving, sighing, sobbing, insomnia, and unpredictable behavior. You may alternate between crying and laughing or tend to hold back tears. Use for postpartum depression accompanied by hysteria and disappointment. Use for anxiety, fear, and restlessness, and loud sighs that indicate anguish when you have difficulty expressing your feelings. For people who experience stomachache or headache after emotional upheaval.

Kali phosphoricum (potassium phosphate): You are anxious, overworked, worried, excited, and oversensitive to pain. You cry easily and may scream during sleep. You may frequently feel cold. You're prone to dizziness, fainting, laughing fits, and poor memory and suffer from anxiety, gloominess, shyness, and nervous exhaustion.

Lachesis (lance-headed viper): For depression from suppressed emotions and during transitions such as menopause. Worse in mornings. For outbursts and irrational jealousy. You're domineering, vicious, suspicious, and talkative. You believe you're being conspired against. You need open air and have a wild imagination.

Lycopodium (club moss): For fear, anxiety, and insecurity. You're overly concerned about what people think of you, fear rejection, and think others are being critical of you. You fear animals, aging, change, and loss of position. For the insecure person who takes anger out on others. You lack self-confidence about new endeavors. You're indecisive and irritable, but when put on the spot, you excel. For an intellectual who is basically a loner yet likes to have someone in the house.

Mercurius (mercury): For sudden anger with a possible impulse to do violence to oneself or others. You're restless, agitated, and have poor memory, lack of concentration, and rapid speech. You're aggravated by many environmental influences and find yourself comfortable in only a few situations.

Natrum muriaticum (common salt): You may dwell in the past, reject sympathy, and become violent if someone attempts to comfort you. You may be sad from failed romance, feel anxious about everything, and experience prolonged grief. You are gloomy and overly sensitive to comments. Use when you are tearful, emotional, or irritable yet practical. You do not want sympathy and desire to be left alone. For chronic grief from having suffered great unresolved emotional pain. You're easily hurt and hold on to grudges and the past. You dislike going to social events where there will be lots of people. May fear birds, snakes, spiders, and insanity.

Natrum sulphuricum (sodium sulphate): For depression following head injuries.

Nitricum acid (nitric acid): You feel anxious and depressed. There may be extreme sensitivity to noise and touch. You may have a chronic, painful problem with one of the body's orifices.

Nux vomica (poison nut): You are irritable and overworked. You can't sleep due to job stress, business loss, or having overeaten. You may be prone to overindulgences in food and alcohol. You have anger and possibly a violent temper and destructive impulses, and are fussy and fastidious over small things. You dislike being contraindicated. You're hurried, impatient, and overemphasize achievement. You're a workaholic, annoyed by noise, persnickety, domineering, short-tempered, and critical. A difficult work period may cause exhaustion and irritability. You're preoccupied with the past, wishing you had dealt differently with a previous experience. May fear insanity.

Passiflora incarnata (passionflower): For general anxiety, obsessive thoughts.

Phosphoric acidum (phosphoric acid): For extreme mental fatigue, burnout. You may respond slowly or not at all to questions. Talking makes you feel weak, and you prefer to be left alone. You're indifferent, silent, and withdrawn because of stress and worry. You may be lazy, drowsy, confused and feel like your head is heavy. Overwork can make you predisposed. Can use for adolescent depression, chronic fatigue, and long-term grief.

Phosphorus (phosphorus): You're fretful and irritable. You first laugh hysterically then cry. You're very sensitive to outside influences. You feel something negative is about to happen. You fear the dark, thunder, ghosts, storms, and solitude. Sleep improves your condition. You may be tall and thin. You're excessively sensitive and have an active imagination.

Platina (platinum): You feel superior, arrogant, and prideful. You live on past glories yet lack effectiveness in the present.

Pulsatilla (pasque flower): You have depression that alternates with a mild, easygoing manner. You're brokenhearted, weep openly, seek sympathy, and may be clingy. Use for anxiety following bad news. For women who can't leave a bad relationship. Fresh air improves your condition, which may include fear of dogs, snakes, and insanity and cause crying.

Sepia: You may feel suicidal and miserable over life. Lacking joy, you feel despairing and irritable. You may cry frequently with no desire to work or change. You were once a loving person, yet now find life impossible. This worsens as the day progresses. You have an aversion to family and friends. For postpartum blues and menstrual-related depression. You dread that something might happen.

Silica (silicic oxide): For shy yet strong-willed people who get anxious about exams, public speaking, and interviews, thinking they will lack in their performance. Capable of working, you may feel numb in your fingers, toes, and back. You're easily fatigued and cry easily. You fear the future and failure, though you often succeed.

Staphysagria (larkspur): Helps ailments caused by repressed anger. Benefits those that hold their temper until they blow up. For those who are easily offended or sharp-tongued. You have low self-esteem and are unable to express your needs. You may have a hard time sleeping and lie awake wishing that you had said or done something different.

Sulphur (sulphur): Ragged and sloppy, you often dwell on religious and philosophical questions. You may be anxious about your soul's salvation and suffer from delusions, yet be too lazy to help yourself. You're slow and often hungry for cold drinks, sweets, and spices. For the know-it-all person or one who is haughty yet philosophical, creative, impractical, or argumentative for the entertainment of it.

Deep Breathing

When we're stressed, our breathing becomes shallow, but deep breathing boosts the oxygen level in your body, making you feel both relaxed and more energized.

Energy breathing from the ancient Chinese practice of qigong does just this by increasing the oxygenation of the blood, tissues, muscles, and organs. Just sit or lie down in a comfortable position. Smile to relax your mind and body.

Place the tip of your tongue gently against the roof of your mouth and breathe in through your nose slowly. When you breathe out, picture any stress changing into smoke as it leave the body. When you are done, take one more deep breath and slowly open your eyes and come back to the world around you.

Meditation

Meditation incorporates deep breathing and takes it one step further. Practicing meditation improves blood pressure, bolsters the immune system, promotes a sense of well-being, and reduces stress and anxiety.

By quieting your thoughts in meditation, you can learn to detach from what is commonly called the "monkey mind," which is your inner dialogue full of judgments and comments about what is going on around you. But when you meditate, you can hear your own inner wisdom, maybe for the first time. Start by meditating for just a few minutes a day. Set an egg timer for two and a half minutes and focus on your breath, either sitting or lying down.

1. Sit in a comfortable position and close your eyes.

2. Allow your breath to fall into a natural rhythm.

3. Settle your attention on your breath for two-and-a-half minutes or longer. When finished, slowly open your eyes and gently reenter your day.

Yoga

Yoga, which is the combination of breath with movement, is a powerful antidote to stress and a way to "be" in the present moment. Yoga postures also have a direct effect on health, helping to remove toxins and improve nourishment of the cells and reducing blood pressure, anxiety, and stress. Yoga also helps you to befriend your own body, accepting it as it is. This in turn helps you to accept life on its own terms instead of the way you wish it could be. Without this conflict, life becomes more peaceful.

Yoga Nidra

Yoga nidra, or yogic sleep, is the easiest yoga you'll ever practice, since it's done while you are sitting or lying down. It's also deeply relaxing and healing. By listening to either a teacher or a CD, you're led through a guided meditation that helps you access the koshas, or states of mind and body that enhance psychological, physical, and spiritual health and well-being. These koshas include the physical body of sensation and the bodies of breath and energy, feelings and emotions, thoughts, and joy. The more you practice yoga nidra, the more you'll experience its benefits.

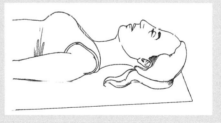

The Relaxation Response

By regularly practicing the relaxation response pioneered by Herbert Benson, M.D., at the Benson-Henry Institute for Mind Body Medicine at Massachusetts General Hospital in Boston, you can reduce stress and feel better. You can elicit the relaxation response in many different ways, including progressive muscle relaxation, diaphragmatic breathing, repetitive prayer, visualization, and guided imagery. In progressive muscle relaxation, you just think of each body part, flex, and then relax it. Start with your face and move downward through your whole body, from your shoulders to your toes. Do it once or twice a day for ten to twenty minutes on a regular basis for best results. For more information, go to www.bensonhenryinstitute.org.

The Power of Now

Worrying about the future and fretting about the past is guaranteed to stress you out. Instead, take the advice of Eckhart Tolle, the author of *The Power of Now*, and stay in the present moment, then act. He writes, "Wherever you are, be there totally. If you find your here and now intolerable and it makes you unhappy, you have three options: remove yourself from the situation, change it, or accept it totally."

An easy way to center yourself in the present moment is by focusing on your breathing. You'll find that much of your stress and fear fades away. For more information, visit www.eckharttolle.com. Sign up for his weekly Present Moment reminder and your email inbox will become an oasis of calm!

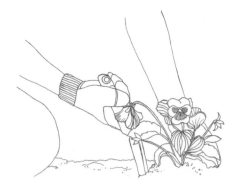

Relax in the Garden

If you have a green thumb, or would like to, spending time in the garden is one of the most enjoyable and effective ways to reduce stress. Plants reduce blood pressure, increase concentration and productivity, and help recovery from illness. A study done at Utsunomiya University in Japan showed that working with plants helps lower fatigue and bring calm. The participants were in one of three groups: filling pots with soil, transplanting nonflowering pansy plants, or transplanting flowering plants. Gardening with flowering plants proved to be more positive than working with nonflowering plants.

Good to Grow!

If you lack outdoor space, the EarthBox (www.earthbox.com), a self-watering patio container garden, is an easy way to grow flowers or vegetables. You can also become a member of a community garden in your town.

Start simply by just looking at plants outside your window or a vase of flowers. Next, add houseplants and then move outside in the spring to garden. Remember, gardening is an affirmation for a fruitful future!

The Power of Negative Ions on Stress

Walking is an effective antidote to stress and even more so if you do it on the beach or in the forest. That's because negative ions, which are found in nature, lower oxidative stress and influence inflammatory chemicals in the body that affect your mood.

No one is exactly sure why negative ions work the way they do, but the theory is that they are generated when water collides upon water. When waves crash or water flows down from a waterfall onto rocks, a "splitting" occurs, creating a higher content of negative ions in the air.

So breathe deep! You can also tap this soothing effect from desktop fountains and from negative ion boxes, which you can put in your home or office.

Find Peace with a Slow Hobby

Slow hobbies such as knitting, painting, sculpting, crocheting, or quilting have a meditative quality that can reduce stress and can help you to relax, along with improving focus and concentration. According to the most recent Craft Yarn Council of America research, 64 percent of knitters and crocheters use these crafts to help them reduce stress and relax. Studies show that these hobbies help to lower heart rate and blood pressure. How do you find the right slow hobby for you? Choose something you really enjoy to put this remedy into practice.

Write It Down

Keeping a journal of your daily experiences can help you to learn what triggers you and what you need to change to be more peaceful. Just putting pen to paper and releasing your troubles is therapeutic. Try this exercise to get started:

1. Make two lists: one of the stresses in your life you can change, the other of the stresses you can't.

2. Rate them on a level of one to ten, with ten being the highest.

3. Write down possible solutions.

 ## Holistic Therapies

Massage helps reduce stress by bringing the body back to its natural rhythm. Regular massage relieves tension in the fascia and improves circulation, which increases nutrients and oxygen to the cells, bones, muscle tissues, and organs and helps remove waste products. Just the act of being touched is good for your spirit, too. Why not get together with a friend for tea and exchange foot rubs?

Reflexology, which focuses on stimulating nerves on the feet, hands, and ears, is also profoundly relaxing. The premise is that pressure points in these areas correspond to other areas of the body, and that reflexology assists the self-healing process by balancing life energy, or qi, in the body.

Acupressure, like acupuncture, focuses on meridians in the body and releasing any blockages that prevent the healthy flow of energy. Try these acupressure points to relieve stress:

LI 4: On top of the hand in the hollow between the thumb and forefinger

UB 10: Where the skull meets the neck on either side of the spine

Yin Tang: Third eye point

Ht 7: The hollow next to the bone on the crease of the wrist in line with the pinkie

 Try these tips to reduce stress and make you more serene each day:

1. Exercise to improve respiration and circulation, send nutrients to the cells, and stimulate endorphin production.

2. Give yourself a massage. Focus on your hands, face, and feet.

3. Reach out to someone. Hug your child, love your mate, lend a hand to a friend in need, or even stroke your pet.

4. Remember to breathe more deeply and slowly. Oxygen nourishes the brain. Alternate nostril breathing is an excellent technique.

5. Slow down your eating, talking, walking, and driving. Do whatever you need to do, but do it slower. Enunciate. Even speaking more calmly can have a soothing effect.

6. Psychotherapy can be essential for releasing pent-up feelings from your body.

7. Some people find that wearing blue and green is calming. Avoid yellow, as it contributes to anxiety. Wear breathable, comfortable clothing that allows freedom of movement.

8. Try a relaxing bath. Light a candle; add a few drops of essential oils such as chamomile, lavender, melissa, or rosemary to the bath water. Soak and enjoy. When done, let the water run down the drain and visualize all your stress going with it.

9. When choosing music, select that which is calming and contemplative.

10. Prepare your clothes, paperwork, and perhaps lunch the night before, rather than starting your morning in a frenzy.

11. Look your best. This is a great way to boost your confidence in all of life's situations.

12. Get out of bed fifteen minutes earlier to allow time to take care of what's needed.

13. Rather than letting your mind carry around so much, get an engagement book and write down numbers, errands, and appointments.

14. Take care of unpleasant or difficult tasks early in the day, so the rest of the time can be spent more easily.

15. Learn to say no to the things you really don't want or have the time to do.

16. Get rid of clutter, which causes confusion.

17. Tell people you need to think about a request before signing up with a yes as a way to manage your time.

18. Practice visualization. There are many CDs and digital downloads available to help you close your eyes and visualize yourself . . . floating on a cloud, lying by a trickling brook. Visit these tranquil places in your mind.

19. Learn to do a craft. Playing with clay is especially stress relieving. To create things of beauty is great for self-esteem.

20. Get a set of Chinese hand balls, available at many natural food stores. Learn to use them.

21. Be prepared for lines that keep you waiting. Have something to read so you don't have to feel like you are wasting time.

22. Smile. Relaxing your face helps the rest of your body as well as putting at ease those around you.

23. Talk to a sympathetic listener.

24. Enlist the help of others. Delegate. You don't have to do everything yourself.

25. Read books that are uplifting. Try *The Urantia Book*, the Bible, or *Tao Te Ching*. Be careful where you put your consciousness.

26. Spend time basking in the beauty of nature.

27. Watching fish in an aquarium is relaxing.

28. Every day, do something you really enjoy.

29. Act like a kid. Throw a Frisbee. Read fairy tales.

30. Spend time in the beauty and quietude of Nature. Go outside and look at the sky. Sit by a stream.

31. Do something for someone who is less fortunate than yourself.

32. Take things one at a time.

33. Pray for guidance.

34. Meditate.

35. Take a short nap when you can. Use earplugs or a white noise machine to ensure quiet.

36. Don't assume that the success or failure of your children is all the result of your influence.

37. Spend quality time with people you care about.

38. Have more fun.

39. Have some alone time every day.

40. Remember that you don't need to be perfect.

41. Get in touch with an old friend.

42. Plan something to look forward to.

43. Remember to count your blessings!

Chapter 3

EASE ANXIETY

Do not anticipate trouble or worry about
what may never happen. Keep in the sunlight.
—Benjamin Franklin

Making room for more joy and happiness in your life means learning how to manage uncomfortable emotions such as anxiety more effectively. Natural remedies and practices can help you to deal with and soothe your anxiety and clear the way for a more peaceful, well-balanced you.

What Is Anxiety?

The word *anxiety* comes from the Latin *angustia*, meaning "narrowness, restriction, or difficulty." It's an apt description, because when we feel fearful, our world constricts. Anxiety can be a warning of impending pain or potential danger, making us more aware, as this planet can be a perilous place. It can also be provoked by fear of the known or unknown and can occur when we are out of harmony within ourselves or with the people and things around us.

Why Are You Anxious?

In reality, anxiety is unrelated to any real, imminent danger. It is an overreaction of the autonomic nervous system, where the flight-or-fight mechanism is activated and exaggerated, and is usually accompanied by a rush of adrenaline that offers an edge in dealing with an adverse situation or person, by either running or fighting.

Heredity; trauma while in utero; difficult birth or childhood; blood sugar; glandular, respiratory, and digestive disorders; major stress; physical illness; or medication can all contribute to anxiety.

Research indicates that a biochemical imbalance in the amygdala (the alarm center, located in the emotional center of the brain) can cause this psychological imbalance. It's not unusual to suffer from anxiety and depression.

Excess copper in one's body (from pipes or cookware) can be a contributing factor in anxiety. Yeast overgrowth can contribute to anxiety, and anxiety contributes to yeast overgrowth. In Ayurvedic medicine, anxiety is considered an imbalance of *vata*, or the air element.

Symptoms of Anxiety

Anxiety can feel like you've had way too much coffee, like a swarm of bees is buzzing around you or an electrical charge is running throughout your body. Regardless, it's very uncomfortable! Other symptoms can include clammy hands, rapid heartbeat, muscle tension, nausea, stomach distress, and shallow, rapid breathing resulting in excess carbon dioxide, which can make you feel light-headed, dizzy, numb, tingly, or sweaty; you may experience chest pain.

Long-Term Effects of Chronic Anxiety

Chronic anxiety can increase the risk of heart attack, precede an asthma attack, worsen diabetes, and weaken immunity, making us more susceptible to cancer as well as cold, flu, and herpes outbreaks.

Different Types of Anxiety

Anxiety is manifested in different ways. If you always feel fearful, despite what is really happening, you may have **generalized anxiety disorder**.

Having a **panic disorder** means you experience sudden attacks of severe anxiety, which are very frightening and can make you feel out of control.

The attacks are brief, only lasting a few minutes, but can be misidentified as a heart attack because you can experience heart palpitations, shortness of breath, and dizziness. Once you have an attack, you may begin to avoid situations that you think provoke them.

If you have **obsessive-compulsive disorder (OCD)**, you tend to have obsessive thoughts or actions, such as going over your to-do list twenty times, washing your hands repeatedly, or checking and rechecking to make sure a door is locked, in a false belief that it will keep bad things from happening.

Phobias range from a fear of heights to flying and snakes. Post-traumatic stress disorder (PTSD) means you relive past traumatic events over and over again, either in your thoughts or dreams.

 Good to Know!

Low blood sugar, or what is known as a hypoglycemic reaction, mimics the physiological symptoms of a panic attack. Unstable blood sugar level can lead to depression and anxiety. This is why it's so important that you keep your blood sugar on an even keel instead of a sugar-powered roller coaster.

For more information about kicking your sugar addiction and keeping your blood sugar stable, read *Beat Sugar Addiction Now!* and the *Beat Sugar Addiction Now! Cookbook*, both by Jacob Teitelbaum, M.D. Visit www.beatsugaraddictionnow.com.

How Natural Remedies Can Help Ease Anxiety

Necessary Nutrients: Antianxiety Diet

Feeding the brain and the central nervous system with the right foods can help to soothe anxiety. The best antianxiety diet is one that keeps your blood sugar at a steady level morning, noon, and night, because symptoms may worsen when your blood sugar dips. This means choosing lean proteins, whole grains, veggies, and fruit and nixing refined sugars and starches.

You may do best "grazing" all day long, eating four to six small meals and snacks, so carry cheese and gluten-free crackers or nuts, sunflower seeds, or pumpkin seeds in your bag each day. The most important thing is to never get too hungry.

Other foods to focus on include oatmeal and yogurt (unless you're allergic to gluten and dairy), both high in calming calcium. Lettuce also helps calm anxiety. Eating nutrient-dense, grounding foods such as buckwheat, millet, black quinoa, black rice, black sesame seeds, sweet potatoes, and winter squash is also helpful.

The Benefits of Fish Oil on Anxiety

In the first study of its kind, researchers at Ohio State University recently found that the omega-3 fatty acids in fish oil calm anxiety. The OSU study included sixty-eight medical students, half of whom received 2.5 grams of an omega-3 supplement daily, the equivalent of about four or five servings of salmon. A study published in *Brain, Behavior, and Immunity* (November 2011) showed that those who took the supplements had a 20 percent reduction in anxiety and a significant reduction of inflammation.

Use a quality fish oil supplement to get your omega-3 fatty acids. Aim for 1,000 mg of EPA/DHA. Purchase a high-quality, pure fish oil supplement to avoid mercury and other toxins.

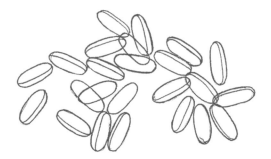

Skip This!

Avoid too much coffee, MSG (monosodium glutamate), stimulants, asthma meds, decongestants, and antidepressants. All drugs and alcohol abuse can trigger anxiety, rev you up, and put your body into panic-alert overtime. Food allergy reactions can trigger a panic attack. Keep a food diary to determine which foods may bother you the most.

Healing Herbs for Anxiety

You've probably heard of kava kava, a plant native to the South Pacific, whose extract has been used for thousands of years in rituals and ceremonies and as a social drink. Kava was given its name by Captain Cook, and it means "intoxicating pepper."

According to the National Institutes of Health, the majority of evidence shows that certain kava extracts (extracts standardized to 70 percent kavalactones) can lower anxiety and may be as effective as prescription antianxiety medications called low-dose benzodiazepines.

Kava kava was recently approved in Germany for its antianxiety effects. You'll need to be patient, though, as it takes up to eight weeks of treatment to see improvement. You'll also need to be under the supervision of a doctor, because this herb can cause liver toxicity.

Other helpful herbs include hawthorn, which nourishes the physical and emotional heart; eleuthero, which helps the body adapt to stress; and California poppy, which is cooling, calming, nonnarcotic, and soothes the emotional body.

Cure Caution:

Herbs such as kava kava can help to ease anxiety, but if you are already taking prescription medications for your condition, check with your doctor before adding supplements.

Wild lettuce extract helps to calm anxiety, while wild oat helps calm acute anxiety. Follow dosage directions on each supplement.

Adaptogens such as ginseng, ginkgo, ashwagandha, and reishi mushroom can also help the body acclimate to stress.

Passionflower targets GABA (gamma-aminobutyric acid), which affects the way neurons connect in the brain. A small study published in the *Journal of Clinical Pharmacy and Therapeutics* in 2001 showed that passionflower was as effective as oxazepam (a medication used to ease anxiety disorders, brand name Serax) for generalized anxiety disorder, without any of the side effects.

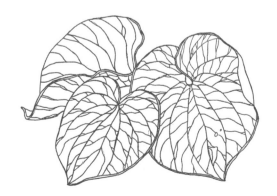

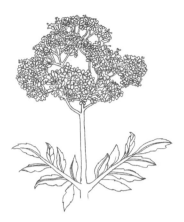

Herbal Teas That Ease Anxiety

Choose soothing herbal teas such as catnip, chamomile, hawthorn, hops, lemon balm, oatstraw, passionflower, or reishi mushroom. Hops and valerian calm anxiety but don't taste pleasant, so try a tincture or capsules instead. When you're feeling anxious, brew a cup of herbal tea and add one dropperful of tincture or take a herbal capsule three times daily between meals.

Well-Being Supplements

A daily calcium (1,000 mg)/magnesium (500 mg) as well as B complex (50 mg) supplement can help calm anxiety. The calming B vitamin inositol (1,500-mg capsule four times daily) that works as a cell messenger is found in our spinal cord, brain, and nerves. Its effect is similar to the drug Librium (chlordiazepoxide) and can help calm panic. Lecithin, eggs, beans, nuts, and avocados are good sources of inositol.

DMAE (50 mg three times daily) is structurally similar to choline, a water-soluble essential nutrient in the B vitamin family. Found in fish and sardines, it protects cellular membranes and transports readily across the blood-brain barrier to calm anxiety.

Amino acids are important when it comes to calming the nervous system and easing anxiety. The amino acid glycine quiets cells in the spinal cord, brain stem, and central nervous system. Taurine suppresses the release of overexciting neurotransmitters such as norepinephrine. The amino acid histidine calms beta waves and promotes more relaxing alpha waves. Amino acids are usually taken as 500-mg capsules three times daily between meals. You can also find combinations of amino acids sold in one pill.

Though you can find GABA (gamma-aminobutyric acid) in passionflower, which helps neurons "talk" to each other and protect the brain from overstimulation, you can take a GABA supplement, too. Many anxious people have low levels of GABA (500 mg taken three times daily, preferably sublingually). Also, 5-HTP (5-hydroxytrytophan) is a precursor to serotonin and is effective against anxiety (150 mg dosage three times daily, preferably between meals).

For Obsessive-Compulsive Disorder

Studies indicate that OCD is often related to a serotonin deficiency. People with OCD often have genetic abnormalities or high levels of histamine. Methionine can help reduce high levels of histamine and is a precursor to adrenaline and noradrenaline.

OCD can be improved with supplementation of inositol, which improves the body's use of the brain chemical serotonin. Talk to your holistic health practitioner about whether this might work for you.

Holistic Therapies: Natural Ways to Calm Anxiety

Homeopathic remedies are a safe and gentle way to ease anxiety. Read through the description for each cure and see which one sounds most like you, then try it. Carry the homeopathic remedy with you and take three to four pellets of 30 c potency dissolved under the tongue three times daily.

Aconitum napellus: You may fear death, darkness, evil, and maybe even crossing the street. Anguish, anxiety, despair, restlessness, and franticness are also characteristic of someone who needs aconite. You may panic in crowded places and fear you cannot get out. Aconite may help with anxiety that occurs when reminded of a disturbing incident from the past.

Argentum nitricum: You may be impulsive and fear impending events, crowds, or heights. Anxiety may precede an interview or exam. You may have panic attacks and diarrhea when anticipating circumstances or get so wound up before an event, your ability to remember what you need to do is impaired.

Arsenicum album: You may be restless, fearful, always in motion, fatigued, fussy, high strung, worried, and fault finding. You may fear death, darkness, and incurable diseases. You may be suspicious and demanding or dislike being in a situation over which you have no control.

Calcarea carbonica: You are anxious about your health and catching infection.

Coffea cruda: For paralyzing anxiety preceding an event such as flying or public speaking.

Gelsemium: For anxiety based on fear, including stage fright or trembling. You are anxious and sluggish and may freeze up physically and mentally before public speaking or an exam.

Ignatia: Sadness leads to anxiety, depression, hysteria, and anger. Use for anxiety, fear, and restlessness; sleeplessness; and loud sighs that indicate anguish.

Kali phosphoricum: You are anxious and exhausted from worrying about relatives.

Lachesis: For nighttime anxiety. You may believe you are being conspired against. You need open air or have a wild imagination. Lachesis is for outbursts and irrational jealousy. You may be domineering, vicious, suspicious, and talkative.

Lycopodium: You lack self-confidence about new endeavors. You're indecisive and irritable, but when put on the spot, you excel. You worry what others think of you, fear rejection, and think others are being critical of you.

Natrum muriaticum: You're anxious about everything, have fearful dreams, or dislike heat, noise, and excitement, which worsen anxiety. You dislike going to social events where there will be lots of people. The condition grows worse with noise or excitement.

Passiflora incarnata: For general anxiety or obsessive thoughts.

Silica: For shy yet strong-willed people who get anxious about exams, public speaking, and interviews, thinking that their performance will be lacking.

How Flower Essences Calm Anxiety

Flower essences work in a way similar to homeopathic remedies. They are made from a "sun tea" (a sun boiling method) of specific wildflowers or trees known for their healing properties, and then diluted. These remedies help to balance negative emotions, freeing the body's energy to heal itself.

In 2007, a study in the medical journal *Complementary Health Practice Review* showed that Bach Rescue Remedy was effective in reducing anxiety. Use the chart below to determine which essence is right for your particular type of anxiety.

How do you feel?	What to take
Generally anxious and stressed	**Rescue Remedy** reduces stress and tension
Worried or fearful about things working out, e.g., money and health	**Mimulus** puts fears into perspective
Fearful and anxious and don't know why	**Aspen** restores a sense of calm and security
Deep-seated anxiety, restlessness	**Agrimony** calms anxiety, makes you feel grounded
Constant low-level anxiety, like a persistent hum	**Larch** restores well-being

Keep flower essences on hand in several convenient places, such as a briefcase, your desk, your purse, and the glove compartment of your car, and use it when anxiety starts to come on. Two drops under the tongue is all it takes. You can also add a few drops of the remedy to a glass of water and sip it slowly. If you are sensitive to the alcohol in flower essences, apply the remedies externally to your wrists and/or temples.

Make Sense of Anxiety with Aromatherapy

Aromatherapy is one of the quickest and most effective ways to soothe anxiety. That's because of the link between our sense of smell and the limbic, or emotional, center of the brain. Inhale the anxiety-relieving essential oils of basil, bergamot, cedarwood, chamomile, cypress, geranium, hyssop, jasmine, juniper, lavender, marjoram, melissa, myrrh, neroli, orange, petitgrain, rose, rosemary, sandalwood, thyme, and ylang-ylang.

If you aren't sure which scent you like best, try several different types and see how you react. Then, when you are feeling anxious, put three to four drops on a tissue and inhale deeply. You can also put essential oils in a diffuser to fill any room with an anxiety-reducing aroma.

Natural Practices
The Relaxation Response

As noted in chapter 2, the relaxation response was pioneered by Herbert Benson, M.D., of the Benson-Henry Institute for Mind Body Medicine at Massachusetts General Hospital in Boston. It is one of the most effective mind-body therapies you can master when it comes to anxiety. Research shows it is a very effective tool for anxiety and medical conditions exacerbated by it, such as migraines and irritable bowel syndrome. By reducing anxiety it stops the excess production of stress hormones such as cortisol and epinephrine. So not only will it calm you down, it will make your body function more effectively as well.

Practicing the relaxation response is simple. You just focus on a phrase or a set of phrases. Doing this reduces the stimulation in the emotional center of the brain, making you calmer. Here's how to do it:

1. Sit or lie down in a quiet place.

2. From head to toe, progressively relax all the muscles of your body.

3. Next, focus on repeating a word, phrase, or image silently to yourself.

4. When other thoughts arise, detach and let them go.

5. Start with ten minutes, twice a day, and work up to twenty.

Good to Grow!

Lavender is a simple plant to grow and care for. Harvest the flowers, make them into a sachet, and place it near your pillow when sleeping to reduce anxiety and induce sleep.

The more you do the relaxation response, the better you will feel. For more information, visit www.bensonhenryinstitute.org.

Yoga Nidra: The Easiest Yoga You'll Ever Do!

One of the most effective, enjoyable, and pleasurable ways to elicit the relaxation response is to practice yoga nidra or yogic sleep. All you need to do is lie down and listen for fifteen to forty-five minutes, every day or second day (but not after a meal).

Research conducted at Stanford University, Walter Reed Army Medical Center, Ohio State University, and others has proven its effectiveness in improving health. A study in the medical journal *Psycho-Oncology* in 2007 showed that guided imagery such as the kind in yoga nidra helps to relieve anxiety. Research is ongoing on the effects of yoga nidra on post-traumatic stress syndrome.

Either listen to a teacher to guide you through the practice or use a Divine Sleep yoga nidra CD. Jennifer Reis (www.jenniferreisyoga.com) has developed three excellent yoga nidra CDs: Divine Sleep Yoga Nidra, Guided Relaxation, and Deep Relaxation. The CDs are available on her website and www.amazon.com.

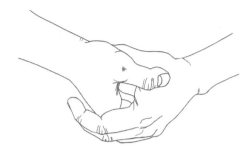

Acupressure

Acupressure is easy to do and provides instant results. Just gently press or rub the space between the eyebrows in the center of the forehead to help calm anxiety and thus, the shen (spirit). Apply pressure to the center of the left palm with the right hand firmly for one minute (where the middle finger ends). Hold the thumb of one hand with the other as a calming technique. Holding your toes, especially the middle toe, helps to bring the energy down from the head and ground it. Repeat as needed.

Breathing

We all must breathe, but conscious breathing can be especially helpful if you suffer from anxiety. When you breathe deeply, you feed your brain the oxygen it craves for serenity. Breathe deeply and slowly and feed your brain the life force of oxygen that it thrives on, calming anxiety. Or try breathing into an empty paper bag (not plastic) for ten breaths to recycle the same air, allowing for more carbon dioxide to be inhaled and calming rapid breathing.

Eckhart Tolle, the author of *The Power of Now,* recommends concentrating on the breath to help move your attention back into the present moment. This can also reduce anxiety, as you are not thinking about the past and what went wrong or fearing the future. As he writes, "Focus your attention on the now and tell me what problem you have at this moment." You may find that nothing is really wrong, right now.

Exercise is also a good way to bring more oxygen into the body and as a result, reduce anxiety. Exercise outside in green places for added benefits.

A study in the *Journal of Physiological Anthropology* shows that walking in the forest and enjoying the benefits of forest bathing, or what is known in Japan as *Shinrin-yoku,* helps to lower the stress hormone cortisol, and gets you out of the fight-or-flight mode. Research published in the *International Journal of Environmental Health Research* also showed the clear effects of "green exercise" on blood pressure, self-esteem, and mood. Negative ions, which have been shown to lower oxidative stress and influence inflammatory chemicals that may alter mood, are also present in the forest, at the beach, and near waterfalls. So breathe deeply!

Prayer, visualization, peaceful mantras, and yantras also calm the spirit. Biofeedback, hypnosis, guided imagery, and sound healing can all be effective therapies to explore in overcoming anxiety.

Art Therapy

Practicing art therapy in the form of drawing, painting, sculpting, or photography can help you to express your emotions and work through anxious feelings. A study in the *Journal of Allergy and Clinical Immunology* in 2010 showed that art therapy helped to reduce anxiety in children with asthma, who had seven weekly art sessions, and for weeks afterward. But it can help you no matter what age you are.

Thrifty Cures

Keeping the kidneys nourished and warm by dressing warmly can help to calm your anxiety and make you feel empowered. Try wearing the color blue. It's tranquil and soothing to the spirit.

In this type of therapy, you'll work with an art therapist by telling her the issues that you are working on, and then you'll be guided through the process of creating as a way to express and resolve how you are feeling. You may find that the process of creating will help you "get out of your own way" and get a fresh perspective, regardless of your skill level.

Learn How to Take Control When Panic Attacks

When a panic attack occurs, stay put, focus on something else, and distract yourself. Remember that however panicked you are, this feeling will pass and not harm you. Breathe, sit, and put your hands firmly on the table; say "STOP" aloud; relax your body and uncross your knees.

Say a comforting prayer such as the Lord's Prayer or a sacred chant or mantra, or count backward from 100 by 3s. Or try focusing on a still object in the room and lose yourself in its details. Describe it over and over and get lost in it. Continue till you feel calm.

Afterward, you can ask yourself what the attack was trying to protect you from. Write about your answers and feelings. Visualize what you want and write about it. Rate the episodes on a scale of 1 to 10.

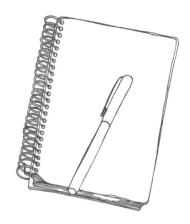

Write It Down

Think and write about what has triggered the past few panic attacks. Are there any common denominators such as a food, place, theme, certain person, or situation? Make a list of the people and places you typically encounter. Ask which of those feel safe and which don't. Put a mark by all those that feel threatening and try to limit those situations. Create a safe space in your home, your work area, and with friends and family.

Rethink Your Routine

To minimize anxiety and prevent panic attacks, avoid the dangerous. When attending situations that cause anxiety, go with a friend, avoid sugar and alcohol beforehand, and be sure to take your calming supplements, such as your B vitamins, before leaving.

Try Cognitive Behavioral Therapy

If your anxiety doesn't respond to these natural treatments, it's time to see your health care practitioner and consider traditional therapy or cognitive behavioral therapy (CBT). This type of therapy is particularly helpful for phobias and is proactive and goal oriented, helping you to identify negative behaviors and thought patterns and then change them so they are more positive. For example, if you have anxiety, you may think, "I am always in danger."

CBT therapists work with you to challenge irrational beliefs and replace them with a more realistic view of reality, for example, "I am safe." You'll be encouraged to write down your anxious thoughts and practice new ways of behaving outside of your sessions.

Research shows that CBT is useful for anxiety disorders, helping to change brain functioning and helping you to be calmer and happier. Ultimately CBT is about taking control of your negative thoughts and changing them to positive ones so you feel happier.

What to Do about Worry

"Worry is like a rocking chair. It goes back and forth but gets you nowhere."
—Mark Twain

Life is uncertain. Worry does serve the purpose of helping us be vigilant and focused, forcing us to act to prevent future problems. But most of the effects of worry are negative. We often worry about things that already happened or may never happen. This can make it hard to think or make decisions, making us less efficient, overwhelmed, and out of control. Worry interferes with sleep, makes us tired and tense, and can cause headaches and stomachaches. Worry also can stimulate adrenaline secretion, thus constricting blood vessels, elevating heart rate and blood pressure.

The Earth Element

In Asian medicine, the emotion of worry is centered in the system of the stomach and spleen and considered part of the Earth element. An imbalance in this element can manifest in obsession, overprotection, and a meddlesome character. It can also make us more prone to laziness and sluggishness.

Overthinking is another aspect of this element. As the mind uses lots of energy, thinking too much can deprive other organs of energy and contribute to poor digestion and a flabby constitution.

Four Ways to Handle Worries

- Rather than focusing on the worry, focus on doing something about it. If you can't figure things out, brainstorm solutions with a trusted friend.

- Stay busy to crowd out worry. Active people don't have time to worry!

- Share your problems with a trusted friend or family member. Tell them what is troubling you. Clear your mind and heart.

- Set boundaries. If you must worry, designate one hour of the day to this activity. When that hour is up, you're done!

Necessary Nutrients

To nourish away the worries, eat Earth element nourishing foods such as millet, hazelnuts, rutabagas, sweet potatoes, and winter squash.

Healing Herbs for Worry

Beneficial herbs to use to reduce worry include the stomach/spleen/chi tonics astragalus, cinnamon, ginseng, and licorice. Motherwort is a beneficial herb for those who tend to "overmother." Passionflower helps calm those with overactive imaginations and calms the mind, thoughts, and worry.

Flower Power

Flower essences for worry include:

Mimulus: For worry that things will not work out, that misfortune will occur and suffering will result.

White chestnut: For persistent unwanted thoughts, preoccupation, insomnia, or nervous worry.

Heather: Helps those who are obsessed with their own problems.

Aromatherapy Aid

Essential oils to help alleviate worry include clary sage, jasmine, and ylang-ylang. Put them in a diffuser or take five to ten deep inhalations right from the bottle!

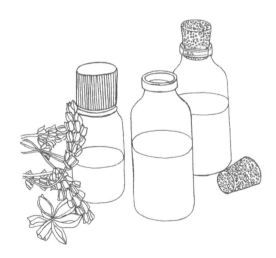

Journaling

If worry persists, consider taking the last five minutes of every hour to write down what is worrying you in order to identify the problems.

Separate problems into categories, for example, home, family, work.

Next, ask what you can do about each worry right now.

If you can take action, break the problems down into smaller steps and take one step at a time.

Journal on this topic: "What is the worst that can happen?" Once you know what that is, chances are you'll be able to face the possibilities with more sanity.

Replace things you often have heard yourself say, such as, "I should" or "I can't," to "I choose," "Let's try," "Why not?"

If you can't take action right now, use the **Serenity Prayer:** God grant me the serenity to accept the things I cannot change, the courage to change the things I can, and the wisdom to know the difference.

When to See Your M.D.

Although these natural remedies can help to ease your anxiety and worry, see your health practitioner if your anxiety is significantly affecting your day-to-day living. These natural cures are not a substitute for proper medical care. With more serious disorders such as phobias, generalized anxiety disorder, panic attacks, or OCD, you may need a combination of therapy and prescription medications to function more effectively.

Good to Know!

Many of the practices in chapter 2 can also help you to relax and let go of worry. Try them!

Chapter 4

ENHANCE MOOD

Have patience with all things, but chiefly have patience with yourself. Do not lose courage in considering your own imperfections but instantly set about remedying them—every day begin the task anew.
—Saint Francis de Sales

Depression is more than having an occasional "off day" when things just aren't going your way. It's a pervasive mood that ranges from a mild case of the blues to a black cloud that follows you around. Depression can affect every aspect of your life, from the way you feel to the thoughts you think, how you sleep, what you eat, and how you interact with others.

Depression harms the vital energy of the body, which can translate into physical symptoms such as paleness, slumped shoulders, sunken chest, weak arms, and a head that juts forward as if reflecting feelings of heaviness.

Many of us have experienced bouts of depression as a reaction to a traumatic event such as loss of a loved one, work changes, an unsatisfactory move, or unwanted changes. You may also suffer from malaise if you're stuck and don't know how to move forward. However, this type of depression is considered a normal reaction and exogenous, meaning due to external factors.

Why Are You Depressed?

If you can't pinpoint the cause of your depression, it may be due to chemical imbalances in necessary neurotransmitters. Low levels of key amino acids such as phenylalanine, tyrosine, and dopamine can cause depression. That's because these amino acids are precursors to mood-regulating neurotransmitters called monoamines, such as serotonin, melatonin, norepinephrine, and dopamine.

Depression runs in families, so if your mother or father suffers from this condition, you may too. Other factors include hypothyroidism, which means your body isn't producing enough thyroid hormone, and conditions such as chronic fatigue, fibromyalgia, and Lyme disease.

Certain drugs can make you more prone to depression, such as progesterone, estrogen, cortisone, barbiturates, amphetamines, and L-dopa. Depression can be aggravated by food allergies and sensitivities that cause cerebral inflammation. Depressed people often have digestive disorders, including constipation.

To be diagnosed with depression, one must have at least four of the following symptoms for more than two weeks.

- Lack of confidence or low self-esteem
- Pessimism
- Lack of interest in ordinary activities
- Withdrawal from social activities
- Fatigue or lethargy
- Irritability or anger
- Decreased productivity
- Difficulty making decisions
- Insomnia
- Poor concentration

- Overuse of drugs or alcohol
- Crying easily or inability to cry
- Hyperactivity
- Changes in eating patterns
- Untidy appearance
- Guilt
- Excessive weight loss or gain
- Missing work, school, etc.
- No interest in surroundings, pleasure, or sex
- Self-hate
- Inability to get out of bed, oversleeping
- Feeling of numbness
- Suicidal thoughts
- Headache

Once you have your diagnosis, you can begin to put your life back in balance.

It's important to keep in mind that these symptoms can indicate other disorders or health conditions, so you'll need to be evaluated by your own health care practitioner. If you are feeling seriously depressed, even suicidal, see your doctor immediately or go to your local emergency room. Ask for the help of friends and family members. You don't need to do this alone.

For those who have mild to moderate depression, these nutritional and holistic therapies can begin to help put your life back into balance. In fact, Harvard researchers found that more than half of people who have depression and anxiety use alternative medicine to get well.

 Good to Know!

In Traditional Chinese Medicine, depression results from a stagnant condition of the liver. Anger is said to be the result of liver energy rising, and depression is more of an inward sensation in which anger is turned against oneself. How does the liver become stagnant? Stuffing emotions without expressing them doesn't help.

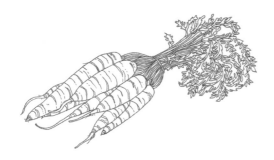

Necessary Nutrients

 Because nutrition affects the structure and function of the brain, it makes sense that healing depression means eating differently. The best diet for depression is to consume small, frequent complex carbohydrate meals that keep blood sugar levels at an even keel.

Lean meat, chicken, eggs, fish, tempeh, and tofu all provide protein, which helps to keep blood sugar stable, and are rich in B vitamins that balance your mood by improving neurotransmitter function. According to a 2010 study in the *American Journal of Clinical Nutrition*, older adults who were deficient in their Bs had a higher risk of depression.

Complex carbohydrates such as quinoa, buckwheat, teff, amaranth, spelt, barley, brown rice, black rice, oatmeal, and millet are digested more slowly, which keeps you off the blood sugar roller coaster. Complex carbs also increase the levels of serotonin, the happy hormone, in your brain. Oatmeal also possesses many healthful antioxidant and anti-inflammatory compounds, including carotenoids, tocols (vitamin E), flavonoids, and polyphenols.

Eat nutritious veggies such as artichokes, burdock root, and carrots. Drink vegetable juice combinations of carrot, celery, watercress, and spinach. Dilute juices with 50 percent water to refrain from overstimulating the pancreas. Use healthful condiments such as onions and scallions as well as ginger, basil, and oregano for flavor. An apple a day keeps the doctor away, and so do all types of berries and citrus fruits. Eating two ripe bananas a day is said to help the production of both serotonin and norepinephrine.

Go Green

Nourish the body with green leafy vegetables such as kale or collards as well as wild greens like dandelion greens, lamb's-quarter, and malva, which are rich in chlorophyll and help transport oxygen into the body. Include mineral-rich sea vegetables such as kelp, dulse, or wakame to nourish the thyroid and boost a sluggish metabolism.

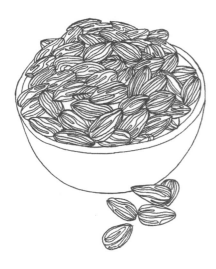

and 400 micrograms of folic acid each day to support nerve function.

Calcium and **magnesium** are essential for nerve and muscle function. Taking 1,000 mg of chelate or citrate calcium and 500 mg of magnesium can help improve your outlook.

Go Nuts!

Cashews, almonds, sunflower seeds, and pumpkin seeds are all high in magnesium, which helps the body produce more serotonin, the happiness hormone, and improves energy. Nuts also are protein rich and help to keep blood sugar stable. Try them as a healthy snack.

Well-Being Supplements

Not getting enough B complex can lead to irritability and mental sluggishness. Folic acid also influences your mood. Low levels of folic acid can also determine whether or not talk therapy or prescription drug therapy is useful. This nutrient even improves how well antidepressants work and helps to minimize side effects. Research in the *Journal of Psychopharmacology* (2005) showed that people who were deficient in B_{12} and folic acid were more likely to be depressed. Take B_{12} (50 to 100 mg)

Thrifty Cures

Foods that are sour and bitter help move liver stagnation. Adding the juice of half lemon to a glass of water helps to stimulate the flow of bile and improve digestion.

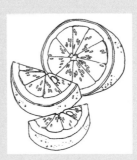

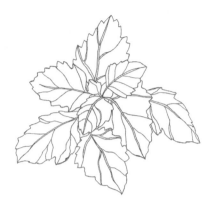

Go Fish!

Omega fatty acids are important because our brains are more than 50 percent fat. Fatty acids help neurons function optimally and increase gray matter, so we can focus and think clearly and also stabilize mood. Eat cold-water fish such as cod, wild salmon, herring, and mackerel three times a week (fish protein also balances blood sugar) to fill up on omega fatty acids or supplement with a high-quality fish oil high in eicosapentaenoic acids (EPA) that is free of contaminants. Folic acid, B_{12}, selenium, and zinc are linked with depression, and all of them influence omega-3, so add these supplements as well.

SAM-E

SAM-e (S-adenosylmethionine) is in every cell, with the highest concentrations in the brain, adrenal glands, and liver, and helps relieve depression by raising the levels of the neurotransmitters serotonin and dopamine and making the receptors for these compounds more available. It also improves energy.

A number of controlled trials have shown that both oral and intravenous SAM-e are of value in the treatment of mild to moderate depression. A 2002 review by the Federal Agency for Healthcare Research and Quality revealed that SAM-e was more effective than a placebo at relieving depression. If you have bipolar disorder, don't take this supplement without discussing it with your doctor.

DLPA

DLPA (DL-phenylalanine) works to heal depression in two ways. It stimulates endorphin, norepinephrine, and noradrenaline production and inhibits the enzymes that break down the body's natural feel-good endorphins to survive longer. It works best if you have depression coupled with low energy, a sense of helplessness, and low self-esteem. It can also help if your blues are the result of change, like the loss of a loved one. It has also been found to benefit the depressive phases of bipolar depression, depression with schizophrenia, PMS, and the depression resulting from drug withdrawal.

L-tyrosine, a precursor for the happy hormone serotonin, can be helpful for those with too little noradrenaline or dopamine brain activity. Take 500 mg in the morning and midafternoon. Tryptophan, an amino acid that helps the body produce serotonin, can help lift depression.

Skip This!

Avoid tyrosine and tryptophan if using MAO-inhibiting drugs, or if following a diet where you must limit your intake of the amino acids phenylalanine, tyrosine, tryptophan, or histidine.

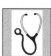

When to See Your M.D.

If you are already taking antidepressants, talk to your doctor before switching to Saint-John's-wort. This herb also can effect and interact with other prescribed medications, such as birth control pills, drugs used to control HIV infection, anticancer drugs, and drugs that help prevent organ rejection. It can also make you more sensitive to sunlight.

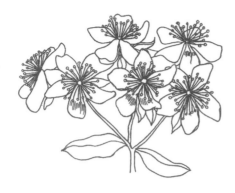

Healing Herbs

Herbs offer a safe and healthful alternative to prescription medications without side effects. However, if you are on medication, do not stop taking it abruptly or add herbal remedies without getting your doctor's approval. Using both at the same time may have unpredictable results. Some herbs that help improve depression follow. Use one cup of tea, one dropperful of tincture, or two capsules, three times daily.

Dandelion root: Improves liver function by stimulating bile production.

Eleuthero: Helps you better cope with stress. It relieves depression, fatigue, insomnia, and stress.

Ginkgo biloba: Improves circulation and helps the brain utilize oxygen better, which can help elevate mood and memory. Increases cellular glucose uptake and improves neural transmission. Helps preserve omega-3 fatty acid levels to improve mood.

Kava kava: Good for easing mild depression and anxiety.

Lavender: Its uplifting aroma helps alleviate fear, anxiety, exhaustion, and depression.

Lemon balm: Traditionally used for melancholy, depression, anxiety, and coping with difficult life situations. The famous Arabian physician Avicenna said of this herb, "It causeth the mind and heart to be merry." It acts upon the autonomic nervous system, protecting the brain from excessive external stimuli.

Licorice root: Helps to keep blood sugar levels stable. One variety of licorice (Glycyrrhiza uralensis) has been found to have an MAO-inhibiting effect 450 times stronger than the drugs used.

Motherwort: Traditionally used for anxiety, depression, exhaustion, gloom, and overworry.

Oatstraw: Rich in nerve-nourishing nutrients. It aids convalescence, debility, drug addiction, exhaustion, insomnia, and post-traumatic stress.

Rhodiola: Good for improving mild to moderate depression.

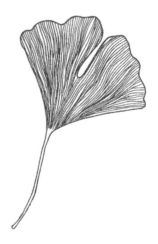

Saint-John's-wort: A popular natural remedy for mild depression. It acts in a similar way to selective serotonin reuptake inhibitor antidepressant drugs, or SSRIs, such as Prozac. Research suggests that a Saint-John's-wort supplement taken once a day may be as effective as the prescription drug sertraline (Zoloft) for people with mild to moderate depression. This herb inhibits both A and B monoamine oxidase, slowing down the breakdown of neurotransmitters norepinephrine and serotonin, and is rich in flavonoids and amino acids such as glutamine and lysine. Unlike prescription medications, it doesn't have side effects such as dry mouth, nausea, headache, or sexual dysfunction.

Ancient Chinese Wisdom

Hsiao Yao Wan, also known as Bupleurum Sedative Pills, or **Free and Easy Pills**, help to improve liver stagnation, irritability, and depression. This formula encourages the free-flowing energy of the liver, thus improving circulation and easing stress. Da Chai Hu Wan or Great Bupleurum Pills are specific for those with severe depression and a tendency to constipation. Find these pills in natural health food stores.

Natural Practices

Many natural practices such as yoga, homeopathy, aromatherapy, and flower essences can help to alleviate a blue mood or mild depression.

Homeopathic Remedies for the Blues

Homeopathy is the practice of like treating like. You'll find the name of the homeopathic remedy in bold and after that a description of the condition it treats. Find the condition or state of mind that is the closest to the one you are experiencing and try that homeopathic cure. Remember: These remedies are not a substitute for care from your doctor or therapist if you are moderately to severely depressed. Talk to your doctor about what is right for you.

Arsenicum album: If you are fussy or obsessively worried about the past, your mind is never at rest, and you toss and turn when sleeping, this may be for you. Also appropriate if you are overanxious, fearful and restless, agitated, depressed, and want everything to be just right.

Aurum metallicum: You feel devalued, sullen, and brooding. For depression following business failure or personal loss.

Capsicum: You dwell in the past; feel homesick, irritable, or depressed; or want to be somewhere else. An overly emotional person, you may feel threatened by new life situations.

Causticum: For depression due to the death of a parent or friend. You feel negative and anxious. You cry over small things and feel gloominess or anxious foreboding that something is about to happen.

Gelsemium: Paralyzed with grief following a loss, you may tremble but can't cry. For mild depression following illness such as the flu.

Ignatia: For acute loss such as that of a child, parent, friend, or pet. Use for grieving, sighing, sobbing, and unpredictable behavior.

Lachesis: Use for depression from suppressed emotions and during transitions such as menopause. For depression that is worse in mornings.

Natrum muriaticum (common salt): Use when tearful, emotional, or irritable yet practical. You do not want sympathy and desire to be left alone. For chronic grief from having suffered great unresolved emotional pain. You are easily hurt and hold on to grudges and the past. You may appear cool and aloof in order to avoid sharing sorrow. You are similar to an ignatia person but may have suffered repeated losses.

Natrum sulphuricum: For depression following head injuries.

Nitricum acid: For when you feel anxious and depressed or are sensitive to noise and touch.

Pulsatilla: Depression alternates with a mild, easygoing manner. You are brokenhearted, weep openly, and seek sympathy.

Sepia: Lacking joy, you feel despairing and irritable. You may cry frequently but with no desire to work or change. This gets worse as the day progresses. You are averse to family and friends. Sepia helps postpartum blues and menstrual-related depression.

Silicea: Capable of working, you may feel numb in your fingers, toes, and back. You are easily fatigued and cry easily. You are melancholy, with difficulty concentrating.

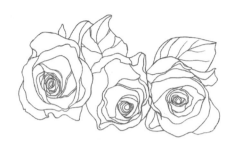

The Power of Flower Essences

Flower remedies help to heal emotional imbalances, such as a blue mood or mild depression. Flower remedies can be taken with herbs, homeopathy, and medications and are safe for people of all ages. Try:

Agrimony: For those who hide their depression with a cheerful facade as well as with drug and alcohol use.

Blackberry: Benefits depression resulting from the loss of a loved one.

Borage: Makes you feel happier. Helps uplift a heavy-feeling heart.

Crab apple: For feelings of uncleanness.

Gentian: Helps with discouragement from setbacks, hopelessness, or despair; for those who are easily discouraged.

Gorse: For hopelessness, despair, despondency, or feelings of inevitable trouble.

Hornbeam: For when you're blue, gloomy, or mentally fatigued.

Mustard: For sudden depression with no known cause. Depression may also suddenly lift.

Star of Bethlehem: For trauma, grief, and loss.

Sweet chestnut: For anguish, bereavement, hopelessness, and despair. Feels like you have reached your limits of endurance.

Aromatherapy

Essential oils that can help lift one's spirits include basil, bergamot, cedarwood, chamomile, cinnamon, clary sage, clove, coriander, geranium, grapefruit, lavender, jasmine, marjoram, melissa, neroli, orange, palmarosa, patchouli, peppermint, rose, rose geranium, rosemary, rosewood, sandalwood, spruce, tangerine, thyme, vetiver, ylang-ylang, and wintergreen.

Put the essential oil or oils in a diffuser and fill your bedroom or office with a soothing scent. Put a few drops on your pillows so you inhale the scent as you go to sleep. Shower with an aromatherapy soap. If you're feeling brave, end your shower with cold water to feel invigorated!

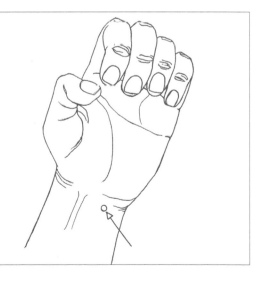

Holistic Therapies
Craniosacral Therapy

Osteopathic physician and surgeon John E. Upledger developed craniosacral therapy in the 1970s to help ease physical, mental, and emotional stress in the body and restore emotional balance. The practitioner does this by monitoring the rhythm of the cerebrospinal fluid as it flows through the system and releasing any restrictions. To find a craniosacral practitioner near you and for more information, visit the Upledger Institute at www.upledger.com.

Emotional Freedom Techniques

Emotional Freedom Techniques (EFT) is a psychotherapeutic practice that can help to relieve depression. The practitioner taps on energy meridian points to release negative emotions from the body's energy field and bring the body back into balance. Visit www.emofree.com for more information.

Mother Nature's News

Acupuncture is a promising treatment for depression in women, who are more prone to this condition. University of Arizona researchers studied 38 women with mild to moderate depression and found that, after 12 sessions, 70 percent of women experienced at least a 50 percent reduction in symptoms, which is comparable to the success rate of psychotherapy and medication.

Acupressure

Try these acupressure points either as part of a massage or by themselves. Apply pressure three times for ten seconds each, several times daily.

1. Press the point 1½ inches (3.5 cm) below the navel.

2. Press right below and on the inside corner of the fingernail of the middle finger.

3. Press directly below the inside corner of the nail of the pinkie finger.

4. Place four fingers into the hollow at the base of the skull. Pushing firmly, massage slowly in a circular motion for three minutes.

5. Apply pressure between the first, second, and third thoracic vertebrae.

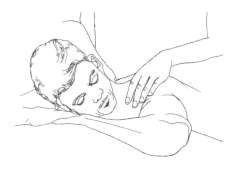

Massage

Getting a massage once a week is more than a luxury; it improves circulation and removes blockages in the body. Try a whole-body massage, preferably using one of the essential oils mentioned above. If you're feeling blue, ask the practitioner to pay special attention to the back of your neck, ears, face, chest, shoulders, legs, and feet.

Exercise

Exercise wakes up the body and stimulates endorphin production, which can mean a happier you. Researchers at the University of Toronto found that moderate exercise can even prevent depression from occurring.

The study published in the *American Journal of Preventive Medicine* in 2013 reviewed more than twenty-six years of research findings and discovered that even low levels of physical activity, such as walking and gardening, for twenty to thirty minutes a day can ward off depression in all age groups.

Exercise also boosts your intake of oxygen, an important nutrient so your brain feels alert, happy, and calm. Smoking, shallow breathing, poor posture, and lack of fresh air all contribute to the brain lacking oxygen. Doing yoga and tai chi and walking outside are all ways to take more oxygen into your system.

Mother Nature's News

Researchers at Boston University School of Medicine and McLean Hospital in Belmont, Massachusetts, found that practicing yoga produced increased GABA (gamma-aminobutyric acid) levels, which can help ease depression. The effect was similar to treatment with antidepressants. Yoga poses for depression include cobra, camel, headstand, and shoulder stand.

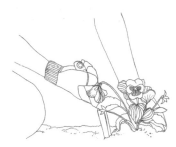

Keep Your Hands Busy, Too

It's been said that "Art is toxic discharge." Sew, knit, clean, work with wood, sketch, garden, paint. Not only will it help alleviate depression, but it will bolster your self-esteem.

Journal Topic

It's time to put pen to paper or fingers to the keyboard. Writing about the way you feel can change your perspective and make you feel better.

Label what it is you've lost (job, promotion, lover, etc.) rather than "everything." Make a list.

Look at the problems as tests and learning experiences. Give your problems a more friendly term. For example, let life's difficulties become learning experiences.

Choose ten activities to accomplish every day (even if it is as simple as getting dressed and making the bed). Write down what you did each day that was productive.

When to See Your M.D.

Dietary changes and dietary supplements are not a substitute for proper evaluation and mental health care. If depression is not adequately treated, it can become severe and, in some cases, may be associated with suicide. Consult a mental health professional if you or someone you care about may be experiencing depression.

Getting Help for SAD

In the winter, when days get shorter, less light can lead to depression, oversleeping, and fatigue, symptoms of Seasonal Affective Disorder (SAD). These natural therapies can help.

Get a full-spectrum light box. It will give you a dose of sunshine for your pineal gland, which stimulates serotonin and melatonin production and vitamin D.

Use a natural alarm clock. A dawn simulator works on any lamp and simulates the early hours of the a.m. by slowly getting brighter over time.

Keep your blood sugar stable by eating foods that contain proteins, complex carbohydrates, whole grains (which also contain vitamins B_6 and B_{12}, which are important for brain health), and nuts, vegetables (which have folic acid), and fruits that are not dried or in juice form, as they are too sweet.

Try tryptophan. It helps your body make serotonin, the feel-good hormone.

Take your vitamin D. The sun helps the body make vitamin D, but in the winter, you'll need to take a supplement. Take 400 mg.

Chapter 5

REST EASY

Sleep is the best meditation.
—Dalai Lama

Blissful sleep is that recharging, rejuvenating repose in which about one-third of our lives is spent. When we rest, our bone marrow and lymph nodes produce substances that aid the immune system, and much of the body's repair work is done. Yet for many, sleep can be elusive, leaving them exhausted and lacking clarity the next day. The best way to improve insomnia is to change the cause.

Reasons Why You Can't Sleep

What you do, think, eat, and drink can determine whether or not you get the sleep you need. Caffeinated foods and beverages such as coffee, black tea, chocolate, and cola drinks, even when consumed early in the day, can affect normal night sleep patterns. Alcohol consumption can interfere with deep REM (rapid eye movement) sleep. Nicotine is a stimulant, and smokers can take longer to fall asleep than nonsmokers.

Many prescription medications contribute to insomnia, including antibiotics, cold remedies, decongestants, steroids, appetite suppressants, contraceptives, and thyroid pills. Allergies, pain, anxiety, and depression can all interfere with sleep. But sleeping pills can inhibit calcium absorption, are often habit forming, can prevent dreaming, and thus should not be a first resort for sleeping problems.

 Good to Know!

Keeping a sleep journal can help you to track the cause of your sleeplessness so you can figure out what is causing it and find answers.

Necessary Nutrients

Foods such as turkey, tuna, whole grain crackers or bread, nut butter, bananas, grapefruits, avocados, dates, and figs all contain tryptophan, an amino acid that promotes the production of serotonin, a chemical in the brain that induces sleep. Try eating a tryptophan-rich snack an hour before bedtime.

Foods that can actually disrupt sleep because they contain the amino acid tyramine, which discourages the production of serotonin, include cheese, spinach, sauerkraut, ham, sausage, bacon, and chocolate, too, which also contains caffeine. Many of the foods in the nightshade family, such as tomatoes, potatoes, eggplant, and bell peppers also interfere with sleep.

Eating too much sugar will give you a temporary lift, but your blood sugar will dip twenty minutes later. You'll feel drowsy at first, but the sugar will actually trigger a hypoglycemic episode (when your blood sugar drops) a few hours later and wake you up.

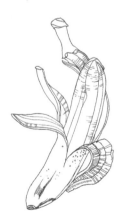

Healing Herbs

Herbal remedies such as valerian can help you drift off to dreamland, naturally. Unlike potent pharmaceuticals, natural sleep cures are usually not habit forming and don't leave you feeling groggy. Here are the ones to try:

Chamomile's antispasmodic properties help you unwind from tension.

Hops contains lupulin, a strong yet safe, reliable sedative. Hops can also be made into a sleep

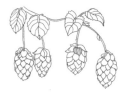

sachet in which a 5- by 5-inch (13- by 13-cm) cloth is stuffed with dried hops, stitched up, and placed in your pillowcase. The aroma from hops helps lull you to sleep. Both King George II and Abraham Lincoln are said to have slept with hops pillows. Make a new sachet twice a year.

Passionflower slows the breakdown of serotonin and norepinephrine, helping you to move into a more peaceful state of consciousness.

Skullcap contains scutellarin, which transforms into scutellarein in the body and stimulates the brain to produce calming endorphins.

Valerian calms sleep disorders that result from anxiety.

All of the above herbs can be taken by themselves or in combination. Natural food stores and pharmacies will carry herbal sleeping blends in tea, tincture, or capsule form. I like tincture or capsules.

If you wake up during the night, place an ounce of water by the bed so that you can squeeze a dropperful of herbal tincture into it. This practice will help you get back to sleep and is simpler than having to get up and make tea, possibly consuming enough liquids that you awaken from the urge to urinate.

Well-Being Supplements

A calcium and magnesium supplement can be helpful when taken before bed, as it has a muscle-relaxing, calming effect. The body also best absorbs calcium when at rest.

B vitamins such as B_3 (niacin) and B_6 (pyridoxine) help produce the body's natural sleep chemicals—tryptophan and serotonin. Take them forty-five minutes before you go to bed; otherwise, they can overstimulate the body's deep sleep cycle (REM) and disrupt sleep.

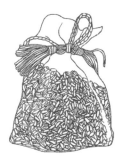

Holistic Therapies for a More Restful Sleep

Essential oils that can aid sleep when placed in the bath or on the pillowcase include chamomile, lavender, marjoram, melissa, neroli, nutmeg, rose, sandalwood, and ylang-ylang.

A warm bath before bed can be a sleeping aid. After the tub has filled, add seven drops of calming essential oil of chamomile or lavender for its relaxing effects. Another technique is to put two or three drops of chamomile or lavender oil on the pillowcase, so you inhale its calming scent when you need to sleep.

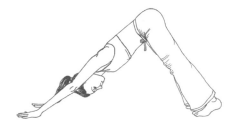

Get Enough Sun Exposure

Sunlight is the most powerful regulator of our biological clock, influencing when we feel sleepy and when we feel alert. So a lack of light exposure can result in difficulty sleeping. If you have trouble falling asleep, spend some time outside in the early morning sunlight, even on cloudy days. Seniors, on the other hand, need light in the late afternoon. Try taking a walk for forty-five minutes or just sit, as long as your eyes are bathed in bright light. If sunlight isn't available, consider a light box or light visor.

Exercise for Better Sleep

Exercise can improve the quality of your sleep. In a study in the *Journal of the American Medical Association* in 1997, Stanford researchers placed sedentary men and women with sleep problems on a program of moderate exercise. After sixteen weeks, the exercisers were getting to sleep twice as fast and sleeping more than forty minutes longer each night.

Although exercise can aid sleep, some studies suggest that exercising too close to bedtime does just the opposite. This is because exercise has an alerting effect and raises body temperature. But if you exercise five or six hours before you go to bed, and your temperature has had time to drop, you'll find you sleep easier. Also, avoid eating at least three hours before bedtime, as food can stimulate rather than sedate.

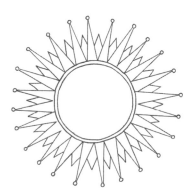

Establish a Sleep Routine

You'll sleep better if you set a regular bed and awakening time and do your best to stick with it. Make the hour to two hours before you go to bed a wind-down period from the day's activities and stresses. Watch television or read in a room other than your bedroom. Try holistic practices such as taking a hot bath or have a massage before going to sleep.

Keep your sleeping environment quiet, dark, cool, and safe for sleeping. The bedroom ideally should be a calm color, such as blue. Put your bed in the quietest and darkest corner of the room. Make your bed as comfy as possible. If you can, use organic sheets and blankets that are as natural as possible to allow your skin to breathe. Set the alarm clock and hide it in the top dresser drawer to prevent the anxiety that can result when you can't sleep and keep checking the clock.

Keep the bedroom between 60°F and 66°F (16°C and 19°C). Allow a bit of fresh air into the bedroom at night, though not directly by the head. Try sleeping on your back because it helps give your internal organs the most room for optimum function.

Make Your Bedroom Allergy Free

Allergies can interfere with sleep and contribute to stuffy noses and headaches in the morning. To minimize allergens wash bedding in hot water (130°F or 54°C) every week to kill dust mites, the microscopic organisms that feed off flakes of dead skin. A dehumidifier, a high-efficiency particulate air filter, and zippered, allergen-proof covers on your bedding and blankets can all help you sleep easier.

Good to Know!

Electromagnetic pollution too close to the body can stimulate the nervous system and weaken the immune system. So avoid having clocks, stereos, and electric blankets as your nighttime companions within 6 feet (1.8 m) of your bed.

Make Your Bedroom a Peaceful Sanctuary

Keep your bedroom space serene and avoid using it as a place to do homework, pay bills, conduct business, or carry out arguments. Avoid excess mental activity right before bed, such as action-packed TV or page-turning novels. Sex, however, can be a pleasurable prelude to sleep.

Dim the Lights

Remember that light is a stimulant. If much light shines brightly through your windows at night, consider getting heavier curtains. If you awake during the night and need to go to the bathroom, avoid turning on bright lights, as this will make you even more awake and inhibits melatonin production needed for sleep. Instead, use a small, red night-light to guide your way. If needed, use earplugs or eye masks to help shut the world out for a while.

Quiet Your Mind

If you have too much on your mind, like plans for the days ahead, things to do, and people to call, write it all down and then let it all go. This makes it easier to relax, rather than needing to lie awake and review your to-do list. If you are troubled about something, try to talk about your feelings with someone you trust.

Focus on Your Breath

When you are ready to go to bed, focus on the in and out of your breath to soothe yourself to sleep. Couple breathing with some sort of visualization. For example, with one breath relax your toes, with the next breath your feet, then your ankles. Moving slowly up your body should help you slumber. By the time you reach your waist you might very well be asleep! Or try counting backward from a high number such as 400, slowly, one number for each breath.

Visualization can also help you to relax and ease you off to sleep. Try closing your eyes and using all of your senses; see yourself in a safe, calm place such as the beach, a lake, or the woods. Or try a CD like Shakti Gawain's Creative Visualization to help you relax and drift off to sleep.

If You Just Can't Sleep

If you can't sleep for more than half an hour, don't fight it. Instead, get up and practice a quiet activity in a dimly lit room that won't rev you up, like reading (no thrillers!), knitting, or listening to calming music until you feel sleepy, and then return to bed.

If you have trouble sleeping, try not to focus on this fact during the day. Just get up in the morning, go through your day, and get into bed at your regular time. Try the strategies you've found here and you will sleep more easily!

Natural Secrets for Sweet Dreams

Dreams are a way of clearing the subconscious and may give us insight about what lies deep in our psyche. It is amazing how in a few seconds we traverse years of experience in these "fantasies of the night." At the very least, dreams can be an opportunity for adventure and entertainment. Dreams usually last from a few moments to more than forty minutes.

Herbs for Sweet Dreams

A dream pillow with an aroma can help access the deep parts of the mind and make dreams more vivid. Make a 4- by 4-inch (10- by 10-cm) sachet filled with dried lavender, lemon balm, and rosemary. Adding a few pinches of ground orrisroot, if you can get it, will help the fragrance last longer. Place the sachet in your pillowcase when you go to bed. Make a new pillow or refill the original every six months.

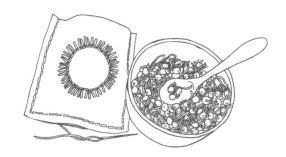

Kava kava is said to induce epic-length dreams worth remembering. Damiana can be smoked or taken as a bedtime tea for vivid dreams. Because damiana is also an aphrodisiac, dreams may be of an erotic nature. Saint-John's-wort is recommended in Europe to promote lucid dreams and help dispel nightmares. Burning jasmine incense before bed may help transport you to the Land of Dreams.

Try sleeping with your head facing north to be in tune with the planetary force fields. The amethyst is regarded as the stone for dreaming. Place some around the head of your bed.

Taking vitamin B_6 (150 mg) and 15 mg zinc before you go to sleep can help dream recall.

The flower essences aspen, rock rose, and Rescue Remedy all help to calm panic and prevent nightmares. Using the color violet in color therapy helps calm the spirit.

Set Your Intention before You Go to Sleep

Before you go to sleep, remind yourself that you wish to remember your dreams. You can also set an intention ("my dreams will reveal wisdom") or ask for guidance on a particular issue. Keep asking. Your final thoughts of the day will often have an influence upon your life. It may be helpful to read something spiritually uplifting before bed to put yourself into a state of exploring consciousness.

 ## Natural Practices for Remembering Sweet Dreams

The best time for dream memories is when you first wake up, but if you begin the day with an adrenaline rush produced by a shrill alarm clock, you'll have little chance of remembering them. Instead, try slowly waking up to soft music or a Zen Alarm Clock so that you have time for reflection. It is also possible to mentally program yourself to wake up a few minutes before the alarm ever goes off.

Once you are awake, try lying still with your eyes still closed. Let the images of your dreams drift into consciousness.

Keep writing implements by the bed to record those flashes of recall. Every morning, write down something about your dreams. If you lack any recall, write, "Nothing remembered." The important point is to get in the habit of writing something daily. Or use a tape recorder or your smartphone to record your memories.

If you can remember a feeling, but not the actual dream, try to think of what situation could bring up that feeling. It may facilitate remembering. Telling your dream to a friend may give you a bit more insight.

Skip This!

Avoid eating before bedtime, as food fuels energy in most cases. Avoid eating sweets after dinner. Excess rich and spicy or oily foods as well as food allergies can provoke nightmares. So can a toxic liver.

Dealing with Nightmares

Nightmares can be disturbing, but they get your attention, and you may want to explore what their significance is. For example:

- Dreaming of drowning or suffocating may indicate the lungs are overactive and need to be calmed.
- Dreams of crying may be an indication of lung deficiency.
- Dreams of failure, such as being unable to complete a task, may mean excess spleen/pancreas energy.
- Dreams of being rejected by loved ones may indicate a spleen/pancreas deficiency.

If the heart system is excessive, dreams of fire, explosives, and heat may occur. A person with a deficient heart may have dreams in which they are unable to talk or scream.

Kidney excess may manifest as dreams of water and snakes. If the kidneys are depleted, the dreams are more fearful, such as being pursued by snakes or swept away by water. Liver excess can result in dreams of impatience, anger, and danger. Liver deficiency may bring dreams of indecision, doom, gloom, and even death.

Herbal Help for Bad Dreams

Banish nightmares with herbal teas and sachets. The ones to use include basil, chamomile, dill seed, rosemary, and wood betony. These herbs can also be hung as sprigs over the bed.

Watching TV before bed can affect your dreams. Watch what you watch! Rather than watching TV in the evenings, you might want to take a walk instead.

May all your best dreams come true!

Chapter 6

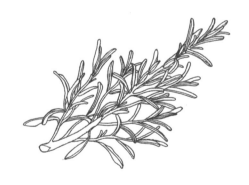

BOOST BRAIN POWER

No matter how closely you examine the water, glucose, and electrolyte salts in the human brain, you can't find the point where these molecules became conscious.
—Deepak Chopra

If you can't remember where you left your keys, or your checkbook or your phone, you're not alone. Nutritional deficiencies; eating the wrong foods and the free-radical damage and inflammation that result; aging; and even conditions such as hypothyroidism and Lyme disease can affect our ability to think clearly and remember important things and can sometimes lead to chronic diseases such as Alzheimer's and Parkinson's. The good news? You can improve the way your brain functions by choosing a better diet for your brain, along with helpful herbs, supplements, and other natural remedies.

How Your Brain Works

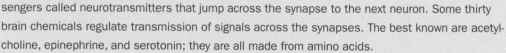

Your brain is composed of about 100 billion neurons, which accounts for almost half of all your nerve cells. Neurons are nerve cells that consist of a cell body (containing the nucleus), a long fiber called an axon (the spinea), and dendrites, which form a tree, like a network of branching neurons.

Neurons never touch and have small gaps between them called synapses. No two neurons or brains are exactly alike, each having its own unique shape.

When stimulated, the neurons release chemical messengers called neurotransmitters that jump across the synapse to the next neuron. Some thirty brain chemicals regulate transmission of signals across the synapses. The best known are acetylcholine, epinephrine, and serotonin; they are all made from amino acids.

Brains will sprout new connections between cells to meet demands as long as our environment challenges or stimulates them. Whenever you learn new things, more links are added between neurons. The saying "use it or you lose it" applies to mind and body! The more you know, the more you can know.

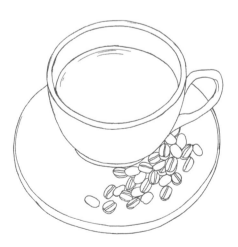

Necessary Nutrients

Foods full of trans and saturated fats contain omega-6 fatty acids, and these encourage the production of inflammatory chemicals called prostaglandins in the body, resulting in free-radical damage to the brain and leading to conditions such as Alzheimer's, Parkinson's disease, ADHD, and depression.

Unfortunately, most of us don't get the antioxidants we need to combat oxidative damage. Research shows that most of us get half of our veggies by eating nutrient-poor potatoes, iceberg lettuce, and canned tomatoes.

Foods that are said to best enhance mental alertness are green leafy vegetables (rich in chlorophyll, which helps the body better utilize oxygen), coffee, flax, walnuts, cauliflower, blueberries (high in antioxidants), and cold saltwater fatty fish like salmon, cod, sardines, herring, and mackerel; are all rich in omega-3 fatty acids. Omega-3 fats are essential because your body can't make them—instead, you have to get them through food or supplements.

Why Your Brain Loves Omega-3 Essential Fatty Acids

Omega-3 essential fatty acids are important because the brain is made up of 60 percent fat. Neurons are also made up of fats and neurological tissue, or what we would call white or gray matter. DHA (docosahexaenoic acid), the most abundant fat in the brain, and EPA (eicosapentaenoic acid) in omega-3 fatty acids improve the health of the cells of your central nervous system and provide structural support, so neurons can communicate. Breast milk contains DHA, which is why it's recommended that babies are breast fed if at all possible.

Good to Know!

Even though the brain makes up only about 2 percent of our total body weight, it requires about 20 percent of the body's total oxygen intake. The brain of a newborn human baby already weighs one-fourth of its adult weight and can grow 1 milligram a minute! By age four the brain has grown to 90 percent of its adult weight, yet the rest of the body is only 20 percent complete in size.

Low DHA levels have been linked to memory loss and Alzheimer's disease, and the older you get, the more you need DHA. A study published in the medical journal *Alzheimer's and Dementia* in 2010 showed that degenerative conditions such as these can be prevented and even reversed. Elderly volunteers who had memory problems showed improvement after taking 900 mg of DHA for 24 weeks.

Other research has shown that DHA also helps with verbal fluency. Even better, when combined with 12 mg of lutein, memory and rate of learning improved.

Skip This!

Food allergies, yeast overgrowth, addiction, and nutritional deficiencies can all contribute to intelligence impairment and memory loss.

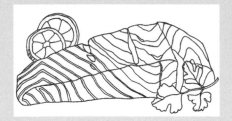

Try This!

If you don't like the taste of fish, get your DHA and EPA in a fish oil supplement. For optimal results, aim for an EPA/DHA amount of 1,000 mg daily. You may also want to try taking krill oil, which, because of its molecular composition, is absorbed much more effectively than fish oil. Plant-based alpha-linolenic acid, an omega-3 fatty acid from flaxseed, walnut, and hemp seed oil that is converted in the liver into DHA and EPA, is also helpful as an adjunct, but go with fish oil first.

Brain-Boosting Foods

The specific foods and the nutrients here can make a difference in brain health by improving mental function, clarity, and memory:

Coconut oil: Your brain is fueled by glucose converted by insulin into energy. If you don't have enough glucose, your brain just doesn't function as well. Coconut oil can help. That's because the ketones in the body that help convert fat into energy (as opposed to glucose) come from medium-chain triglycerides (MCTs) found in coconut oil. In fact, coconut oil contains a whopping 66 percent MCTs. Start with 1 teaspoon a day with food and gradually build up to 1 tablespoon (14 g) daily for maximum benefit.

Green tea: It contains phytochemicals (from the Greek word meaning "plant") called catechins, potent antioxidants with powerful anti-inflammatory properties that prevent damage to nerve cells that is characteristic of such conditions as Alzheimer's and Parkinson's diseases.

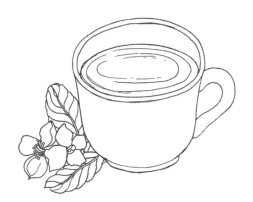

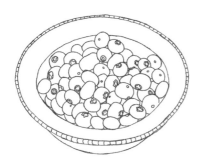

Nuts: Neuroscientists at the University of Illinois-Chicago found that nuts, in particular, almonds, prevent mental decline as we age. Almonds contain good fatty acids like those in olive oil, with plenty of monounsaturated fat. Almonds contain 10 IU of the antioxidant vitamin E (alpha-tocopherol) per ounce and are also good sources of nutrients such as magnesium, copper, calcium, and riboflavin.

Purple and red foods: When you eat blueberries, dark cherries, pomegranates, black grapes, and beets, you tap the power of anthocyanins, strong antioxidants that protect blood vessels, and enhance communication between nerve cells. A study in the *American Journal of Clinical Nutrition* (2005) showed that the phytochemicals such as anthocyanins in blueberries may enhance signaling between nerve cells. Blueberries may also make nerve cell receptors more effective when binding with the brain's chemical messengers.

Green foods: Dark green veggies contain magnesium that lowers levels of C-reactive protein (CRP), a blood marker of inflammation. Their antioxidant properties help protect the central nervous system from the damage caused by oxidation. They also improve memory.

Dark chocolate: This treat is high in antioxidants. Choose organic dark chocolate because it is free from pesticides. It is also lower in sugar, which promotes inflammation in the body.

Sesame seeds: These work as an antioxidant to protect the fats that make up the walls of our cells. Studies show that black sesame seeds popular in Japan are even more effective than white sesame seeds in protecting cells against free-radical damage.

Turmeric: A study in the *Journal of Biological Chemistry* shows that this natural, anti-inflammatory yellow powder found in curry could be an effective enhancer of an enzyme that protects the brain against oxidative conditions such as Alzheimer's disease. You can also take it as a supplement.

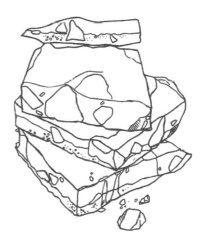

The Anatomy of the Brain

The three portions of the brain are the instinctual (reptilian), limbic (mammalian or emotional), and neocortex (rational thought). The brain stem is the most primitive portion of the brain, evolving even before mammals. It is sometimes referred to as the reptilian brain, lower brain, hind brain, or R complex. The brain stem is actually an extension of the spinal cord. The **medulla oblongata** is the lower half of the brain stem and supports life in many ways, including heart rate, breathing, circulation, and digestion.

Healing Herbs

These herbs have stood the test of time in helping improve brain function and have been used by various cultures throughout history to improve mental capacities. You can benefit from them today:

Ashwagandha supports the nervous system and in Ayurvedic medicine is considered a medharasayan remedy, a promoter of memory and learning.

Bacopa increases attention span and improves behavior, memory, learning, and motor coordination. It enhances learning new tasks and aids in retention of newly learned material.

Eleuthero is nourishing to the pituitary and adrenal glands. It helps the body's ability to deal with stress. Studies done in the former Soviet Union show that this herb helps to improve job accuracy. It improves memory by improving circulation. It is an adaptogen and a chi tonic.

Gotu kola has been used in India as a cerebral and endocrine tonic. Containing calcium, pangamic acid, and phosphorus as well as the amino acid glutamine, this well-renowned herb has been used to treat amnesia, dementia, fatigue, and senility. It has a revitalizing effect on the brain cells and nerves.

The Anatomy of the Brain: The Cerebrum

The cerebrum, which makes up about 85 percent of the brain's mass, is divided into two halves or hemispheres. Each hemisphere contains cellular networks that receive, store, and retrieve information. The cortex is the brain portion responsible for language, memory, and abstract thought.

The hippocampus coordinates information from the cortex to form links (associations) between various sensory representations. The cerebellum (also known as midbrain) houses posture, balance, and movement. The amygdala triggers either aggression or docility depending on the situation and the hippocampus forms and stores new memories.

The Left Brain

The left brain is more analytical, logical, verbal, temporal, and sequential. The left brain controls language, speech, facts, numbers, dates, spelling, linear and logical thinking, reasoning, and analysis; it processes information one step at a time.

The Right Brain

The right side of the brain works more with fantasy, feeling, imagination, and intuition. It's more artistic, holistic, intuitive, musical, and pictorial, and you easily see patterns and relationships and understand metaphor (the difference between what is said and what is meant). The right brain corresponds more to spatial functions such as imagination and intuition, as well as the ability to "see the big picture" and process several kinds of information at once. One way to improve right-brain activity is to think in pictures.

Do you work more with your right or left brain?

Ginkgo helps improve the brain's ability to utilize oxygen and glucose by improving peripheral blood flow. Ginkgo has been found to improve nerve signal transmission and activate ATP (adenosine triphosphate), an organic compound that aids metabolic reactions. Ginkgo helps protect nerve cells from free-radical damage. Ginkgo is currently one of the most prescribed herbs in Europe and is recommended in treating dementia, memory loss, and senility and promoting recovery from stroke. It is an antioxidant and cerebral tonic.

Huperzine, a compound found in club moss, increases brain levels of the chemical acetylcholine and enhances memory, focus, and concentration. It has been shown to improve the cognitive factor in Alzheimer's patients.

Reishi mushrooms help promote mental clarity and peacefulness.

When to See Your M.D.

Memory loss can be caused by hypothyroidism, hormonal changes due to menopause, anemia, chronic Lyme disease, and a vitamin B_{12} deficiency. Ask your doctor for complete blood tests to get the whole picture if you are concerned.

Good to Know!

A Chinese patented medicine for poor memory and inability to concentrate is called **Bu Nao Wan**, also known as **Cerebral Tonic Pills**, which helps with poor memory, loss of concentration, mental agitation, and fatigue. Find it in your local health food store and at Chinese grocers.

Rosemary has a delightful aroma that has a long European tradition of helping to alleviate anxiety. Ancient Greek scholars wore laurels of rosemary when taking examinations, as the smell was found to improve memory. The uplifting fragrance of this member of the mint family is said to stimulate the pineal gland and improve energy levels. Rosemary contains the nutrients calcium, magnesium, potassium, phosphorus, iron, and potassium. Rosemary also contains more than a dozen antioxidants.

Well-Being Supplements

Specific nutrients found in supplements can improve brain function. Look to B vitamins first. That's because the entire **B complex** acts as a lubricant for cellular function, and a deficiency can lead to memory loss and impaired cognition. **Vitamin B$_1$** helps the brain transform nutrients from protein and glucose. It can help mental fatigue as well as memory loss and confusion. A **vitamin B$_2$** deficiency can lead to impaired brain development in the young and behavior problems. Without **niacin**, you may be more prone to depression, short-term memory impairment, and anxiety. **Vitamin B$_6$** helps to produce the neurotransmitters dopamine and serotonin.

Why Vitamin B$_{12}$ Is So Important

Vitamin B$_{12}$ is an essential nutrient in myelin, the fatty sheath that surrounds the nervous system. Low levels can contribute to memory loss. Vitamin B$_{12}$ also helps brings oxygen to the brain cells and reduces inflammation. Highest sources of B$_{12}$ are liver, blue-green algae such as chorella and brewer's yeast. You can also take B$_{12}$ sublingually (under the tongue). Research published in the medical journal *Neurology* (2011) shows that those who don't have enough B$_{12}$ are more likely to score lower on cognitive tests and even have smaller brains!

If you have brain fog or difficulty remembering, you probably have a B$_{12}$ deficiency that needs to be treated. In fact, a study in Finland published in *Neurology* in 2010 found that if you consume foods rich in B$_{12}$, you can slash your risk of Alzheimer's later in life. Fogginess and problems with memory are two of the top warning signs of vitamin B$_{12}$ deficiency, and this is indicative of its importance for brain health.

Folic acid is necessary for the production of RNA and DNA, which is essential for memory and learning and for growth in children. The B vitamin choline increases the brain's rate of metabolism and the metabolism of fats. From this nutrient, the brain makes acetylcholine, which is the most important neurotransmitter involved with intelligence, memory function, and maintaining the structural integrity of the synapses. Acetylcholine diminishes as we age. Choline stimulates its production. DMAE

Learn More about Brain Waves

Alpha brain waves are associated with meditation, relaxation, and detached awareness. Without alpha, you wouldn't remember your dreams. Beta waves correspond to the functions of daily life, when the environment stimulates us, like awakened states, alertness, logical thinking, and problem solving. Delta and gamma waves are associated with inspiration and spirituality. Theta waves are associated with the unconscious mind and the states we encounter in dreaming and meditation.

(dimethylaminoethanol) is chemically similar to choline and helps to make and maintain neurotransmitter function, improves memory, and elevates mood.

Lecithin is used in Europe to treat senility. It helps in fat metabolism. Lecithin accounts for about 30 percent of the dry weight of the brain. When buying lecithin, look for brands that contain at least 30 percent phosphatidylcholine. Both choline and lecithin have been found to be helpful in Parkinson's disease. Human breast milk is much higher in lecithin than cow's milk. The other important component in lecithin is **inositol**, which co-functions with choline as a fat metabolizer and brain enhancer. Vitamin B$_{12}$ can help in the synthesis of RNA.

Phosphatidylserine is a phospholipid that has exhibited the ability to improve memory and cognitive capabilities. It helps maintain the integrity of brain tissue and the fluidity of cellular membranes, thus benefiting neuron transmission. It naturally occurs in brain cells, and amounts tend to decrease as aging occurs.

Vitamin E helps protect the brain from free-radical damage and in turn delays the onset of dementia. Researchers for the Okinawa Program in Japan studied vitamin E levels in Okinawan elders and found that their blood level of vitamin E was 30 percent higher than that of Americans. Elders there naturally eat superfoods such as sweet potatoes and foods that are high in vitamin E like nuts, seeds, olives, olive oil, vegetable oils, avocados, wheat germ, whole grains, and leafy green vegetables. If you don't get enough vitamin E from your diet, supplements can help.

Note: If you take blood-thinning medication, it's very important to check with your doctor before taking any vitamin E supplementation.

A lack of **vitamin C** can lead to hypersensitivity, fatigue, and depression. Vitamin C is also an antioxidant, protecting delicate nerve cells. Vitamin C can be found in fruits (especially citrus) and vegetables, including green and red peppers, tomatoes, and green, leafy varieties like spinach and collard greens. **Note:** Vitamins C and E work synergistically to protect against dementia.

Calcium and **magnesium** are needed for proper brain function. Boron helps to promote mental alertness. **Iron** helps to make neurotransmitters and DNA. Without magnesium we may be more prone to confusion, lethargy, and depression. **Potassium** is needed to maintain normal levels of neurotransmitters. During pregnancy, **zinc** ensures proper fetal brain growth. There is a considerable amount of zinc in the brain.

Beta-carotene and **vitamin A** help carry more oxygen to the brain and help prevent fatigue. Research in the *Journal of Neurology, Neurosurgery and Psychiatry* showed that low levels of **vitamin D** affect brain function. Increasing the amount of this nutrient in the body either through sun exposure or supplementation can help keep you mentally fit as you age.

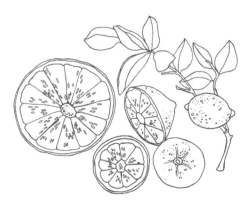

The Peripheral and Sympathetic Nervous System

The parasympathetic nervous system stems from the brain's base, helps in the assimilation of nutrients, contributes to the ability to relax, and is necessary for repair and restoration of the body.

The yin component of the nervous system, it governs internal functions necessary for life support, including breathing and glandular, heart, and digestive activity.

The sympathetic nervous system governs the vital organs, originating from the spinal column. The master branch is known as the pneumogastric nerve, or "abdominal brain," and governs breathing and digestion. The sympathetic nervous system helps discharge previously accumulated energy, burns fuel for work, and aids defense and flight from danger. It responds to emergencies by shutting down nonessential bodily functions at that time. It also regulates stress hormones, sensory response, and heart rate. It is the more yang component of the nervous system and governs the vital organs.

Why Your Brain Needs Amino Acids

Amino acid therapy can improve your mental capacity to enjoy the world. **L-glutamine** readily crosses the blood-brain barrier and becomes glutamic acid. It serves as brain fuel and as a protective agent. **L-methionine** nourishes brain cells and aids choline's ability to promote thinking. **L-phenylalanine** works as a neurotransmitter. It gets converted into norepinephrine and dopamine, which are neurotransmitters that promote mental alertness. **L-taurine** is an antioxidant, an electronic regulator for nerve cells, and chemical transmitter for the brain.

L-tyrosine stimulates the production of dopamine, norepinephrine, and epinephrine, promoting alertness and awareness; it is even mood enhancing and motivating. Low levels of dopamine can contribute to depression, autism, schizophrenia, and hyperactivity. **N-acetyl-cysteine** is an antioxidant that helps to make glutathione. It improves cognitive function, and stabilizes neurological deterioration. **Coenzyme Q$_{10}$** also functions as an antioxidant and decreases from our brains as we age. Consider **octocosonal** for short-term use such as with brain damage occurring from head injury, stroke, or shock.

Acetyl-L-carnitine: An amino acid, vitamin-like compound, it improves memory by stabilizing membranes, boosting energy production, and making nerve transmission more effective. It stimulates acetylcholine production and absorption by the brain.

Ginger: Research conducted at RMG Biosciences of Baltimore showed that extracts of ginger (*Zingiber officinale*) and galangal (*Alpinia galanga*), a member of the ginger family, helped inhibit the manufacture of inflammatory brain chemicals, and in turn slowed down the progression of neurodegenerative disorders such as Alzheimer's.

Natural Practices to Boost Brain Function

Exercise

Exercise increases the body's intake of oxygen and speeds up nerve impulses between brain cells. Studies also show that one hour of exercise five times a week will help prevent degenerative diseases such as Alzheimer's, because it increases circulation, gets rid of stress, and cools off inflammation. Exercise also encourages nerve cells to produce proteins such as neurotrophic factor that improve brain health and cognitive function like learning. Research in the *Journal of Applied Physiology* in 2012 showed that exercise improves the function of mitochondria that produce energy, and in turn brain power.

Supplement Spotlight

Because your gut is your second brain—you even have neurons in your gut that produce feel-good neurotransmitters like serotonin—it's important to keep it healthy. But eating a lot of processed foods and sugar will destroy healthy microflora and breed bad bacteria and yeast. Taking a probiotic supplement can help.

Mother Nature's News

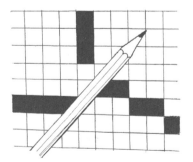

Research in the *New England Journal of Medicine* in 2003 shows that keeping your brain active by doing crossword puzzles, reading books or newspapers, writing for pleasure, or playing board games or cards with friends can help prevent dementia and boost mental functioning.

Choose something that you enjoy so you stick with it. If you love to dance, put on your favorite tunes. If you love the snow, try cross-country skiing. If you love the water, swim. Take a walk and watch the world go by. Aim for thirty minutes of exercise three to four times a week. You'll notice the difference!

Aromatherapy

Because your nasal cavities are very close to the brain, you can use aromas to easily stimulate mental alertness. Try using the aromas of basil, bay, eucalyptus, jasmine, lavender, lemon, lemongrass, lime, peppermint, and rosemary to boost brain power. The smell of vanilla is being investigated for its ability to help people recall childhood memories.

Cineole, which is especially high in basil, ginger, orange, peppermint, eucalyptus, and rosemary, has been found to increase blood flow to the brain. Smell the same essential oil, like rosemary (Greek scholars put garlands of rosemary around their heads and necks to help them learn), when studying and then use it again when taking a test or having to perform.

Aromatherapy can be as simple as putting a few drops of an essential oil on a tissue and inhaling it, putting a few drops on a pillow, or using it as a subtle perfume. Or you can use a diffuser to disperse the aroma into the room.

Holistic Therapies
Acupressure

A good place to massage to enhance mental alertness is the SI-13 acupuncture point, which is found by reaching your right hand over the left shoulder and, with the middle finger, pressing into the pointy edge of the shoulder blade on the upper back. Repeat on other side. This increases blood flow to the brain stem.

Learning about the Limbic System

The limbic system, located on the top of the brain stem, is associated with prolonged emotional responses such as hunger and thirst. Along with the hypothalamus it is associated with human sexual behavior, heat regulation, and the emotions of fear, anger, and motivation. The limbic system is sometimes referred to as the "smell brain," as it is directly connected to taste and smell receptors, which is how aromatherapy works!

Brigitte's Advice for Building Better Brains

Choose things to do that appeal to you or areas you know you need to focus on and take action to build brain power starting today.

1. Expand your experiences. Traveling to school or work by new routes inspires different thoughts as various visions flash by.

2. Avoid being stuck in a rut. Visit new places. Try new foods. Vary the places where you travel for vacation.

3. Hang out with intelligent people. Converse with interesting people. Have a conversation with someone who has different views than you do.

4. Play word games. Have in-depth discussions. Ask questions and get answers, even if you have to look them up yourself.

5. Sharpen your senses by really focusing. Notice as many details as possible. Experience the world using as many senses as possible.

6. Absentmindedness means that the mind was not present or focusing on the matters at hand. Ram Das was right: "Be here now."

7. An ancient saying goes, "I hear and I forget. I see and I remember. I do and I understand." When learning new things, do your best to do it yourself.

8. Practice good posture to better allow the flow of energy throughout the nervous system.

9. Read challenging literature that offers new insights. Try the classics. Enjoy a genre that you have never before read, such as autobiographies, science fiction, or history. Read a magazine with information that is contrary to your own beliefs.

10. Keep a pen or pencil handy. Always have something to write with. You never know when you are going to get a great idea.

11. Make a collage or vision board of what you want to bring into your life.

12. Play with toys. Collect children's toys and get them out to share with your friends. Play!

13. Mozart's music has been shown to improve IQ scores. Chopin, Ravel, and Schubert are said to enhance stream of consciousness.

14. Use your nondominant hand to complete simple tasks such as brushing your teeth, buttoning clothes, and eating. This requires you to use the side of the brain opposite the one you normally use.

15. Use your feet to perform a task like putting clothes in the laundry hamper.

16. Color therapists say that the color yellow is cerebrally stimulating. Highlight important passages that you read in yellow, wear the color, and visualize breathing it in. Consider using yellow in lighting and décor in places where mental work is being done. Full-spectrum lighting elevates serotonin levels.

17. Quietly and closely observe nature. She abounds with beauty and intelligence even in minute detail that can inspire us in a positive way.

18. Free your mind! Write down details—phone numbers, things to do, and goals—to get them out of your head and into action. Keep an engagement calendar. Record flashes of brilliance and words of wisdom. Make lists into meaningful categories.

19. When taking classes, sit in different places to gain different perspectives and foster alertness.

20. When attending lectures, take notes on key words and phrases.

21. When you want to remember something, repeat it aloud to yourself. Visualize it being imprinted upon your brain.

22. To help remember names, associate the name with a picture. Eileen has big blue eyes. Visualize Bob turning into a bobcat. Right after being introduced to someone, use his or her name. "It's nice to meet you, Denise." If you don't quite catch how to say their name, ask them to spell it for you.

23. When learning something important, with your mind's eye, see yourself registering the information and filing it. Then practice retrieving it and re-filing it.

24. Think positively. You'll do better if you affirm that "I can pass this exam" rather than "I'll never make it."

25. Listen to self-help CDs, DVDs, and downloads. Engage your mind.

26. Avoid damaging substances such as cigarettes, alcohol, pollutants, artificial sweeteners, and MSG. Many medications have an adverse effect on the brain.

27. Try studying in the afternoon or right before you go to sleep to remember more. The ideal amount of time to study is thirty-five minutes. In the last five minutes, review what was studied for the first thirty. Take a break in between study sessions if you need to study longer than thirty-five minutes.

28. You may find that recording dreams gives you new insight. While dreaming, the brain generates chemicals and protein needed during awake time. People dream in color but usually remember dreams in black and white.

29. Spend time each day doing nothing. Give the overworked brain time to rest.

30. Learn about mudras (sacred hand gestures), mantras (sacred chanting), and yantra (pictures that help awaken the divine within). For example, chanting the mantra "om" aids opening of blockages in the spinal column as well as stimulating the pituitary and pineal glands.

31. Sleeping with a sachet of rosemary in the pillowcase may help you to recall dreams. Before going to sleep, tell yourself that you want to remember dreams. Upon awakening, give yourself a few minutes to reflect and write down the stream of dreams that occurred. Having a notepad and pencil by the bed may give you the opportunity to record other important thoughts as well.

32. Work in teams. Draw on the skills and ideas of friends and coworkers. Practice the art of brainstorming, where you record wild thoughts and ideas. This often leads to fruitful concepts.

33. Break chains of blockage and negative thought with diversion. Go for a walk. Call a friend. See a movie.

34. Creative people usually retain a childlike quality. My friend Timothy Leary, Ph.D., used to say, "Adulthood is a terminal disease."

35. The art of visualization is one way of practicing mental gymnastics. Einstein supposedly came upon the theory of relativity while visualizing flying along at the speed of light.

36. Meditation is helpful to both calm and expand consciousness. Ideally meditate daily in the same place at the same times. In the morning soon after awakening and before eating are ideal. Sitting on a mat or chair will prevent the inclination to fall asleep. Sit quietly with your hands resting on your lap or gently beside you. Breathe softly, in and out. Listen to your internal sounds; simply focus on your breath.

37. Prayer is when we talk to God. Meditation is when God talks back to us.

38. Play mentally challenging games such as chess or Scrabble. Do puzzles, crosswords, and word jumbles.

39. Make up acronyms. To remember your license plate, create a sentence using words beginning with each of the letters. For example, MRU607 might be Musk Rat Universe 6 oh! 7 (bizarre and whimsical are okay). Exercises to improve memory are called mnemonics, where you make up interesting information to help you remember something. For example, to remember the planets in their order of distance from the sun, take the first letter from each word: Mary's Violet Eyes Make John Stay Up Nights.

40. Use rhyme associations: Thirty days hath September. Mnemonics are words formed from the first letter of each item. For example, if your grocery list says buy apples, bananas, and oranges, you might think of the word BOA.

41. Double a number for as long as you can (2, 4, 8, 16, 32, 64).

42. Experiment with devices that can help stimulate various states of consciousness. I have found the ones that use sound through headphones and light perceived through closed eyes and a special set of glasses to be amazing and versatile, providing states of mind from relaxation to high excitement. Many larger cities have places where you can try the machines in the store and even rent them.

43. Introverts tend to have their most creative time in the early mornings, while extroverts work better at night.

44. Learn two new vocabulary words a week. Use them in a discussion or email.

45. Learn a new fact daily (or use a daily calendar that has tear-off sheet with daily lessons). Read an entry in an encyclopedia daily. It is easier to absorb information if it's gathered gradually than all at once.

46. Memorize at least one great poem.

47. Take an ordinary object and think of ten other ways it could be used. A book might be a doorstop, a writing pad a tool to walk with erect posture, etc.

48. Keep learning things of value for your entire life. Learn new skills such as language, instruments, dance, martial arts, capoeira, or drawing. Take a class at a local community college. Join a book club.

49. Keep things organized. Get rid of clutter and distractions. Learn about feng shui.

50. Create art. Sketching, sewing, knit one, pearl two opens up neural pathways and can create works of beauty.

51. Activate your other senses by getting dressed with your eyes closed. (Lay out your clothes the night before.) Enjoy a meal in the dark or in silence. Wear earplugs when walking to experience deeper levels of silence.

52. Listen to music while you are smelling an essential oil.

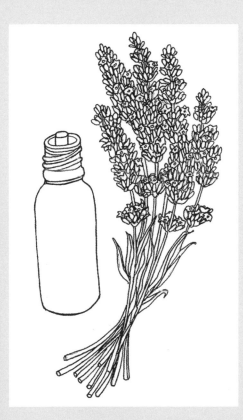

53. Vary the order in which you do things. Shower in the morning instead of at night. Eat breakfast for dinner.

54. Envision a situation and ask, "What if?" Come up with an answer. What would blank do? Fill in the blank with Jesus? Peter Pan? Mae West? Black Elk?

55. Always have a calendar handy. Nowadays many people use phones, but I prefer having it all on paper.

56. Journal Topics:
- Make a list of 100 things you would like to accomplish in your life.
- Make a list of three skills you would like to master.
- Make a list of five things you would like to teach your children.

57. Keep an open heart and open mind. Be open to the possibilities. Remember:

"Necessity may be the mother of invention, but curiosity is the mother of discovery."
—Charles Handy

Chapter 7

MAINTAIN A HEALTHY WEIGHT

To keep the body in good health is a duty . . . otherwise we shall not be able to keep our mind strong and clear.
—Buddha

Tired of battling the bulge? You've got plenty of company. Thirty-four million Americans are at least 20 percent over their ideal weight, which can contribute to a wide variety of problems, including heart disease, hypertension, gallstones, diabetes, lethargy, prostate enlargement, fibroids, and breast, rectal, and colon cancers.

Excess Pounds Burden the Entire Body

To experience this effect, try carrying around a 5-pound (2.3-kg) bag of flour for a few hours. Blood, which would normally reach the brain and provide energy, remains in the abdominal cavity when the body is overburdened.

The heart must work harder and can get weaker and more prone to collapse when you are overweight. Excess weight can stress the spine, knees, and joints, causing pain. Overeating and its resulting excess fats, carbohydrates, and protein can obstruct the blood and be a factor in high blood pressure.

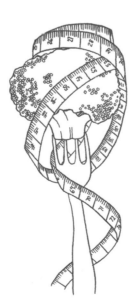

Go Natural

If you're wondering whether you need to lose weight, get naked and take a good look in a full-length mirror. It's supereasy to ignore what you can't see. But don't be discouraged if you are carrying around extra weight; instead, let this practice motivate you. Visualize yourself as you want to look and take the steps that will help you achieve your goals. Start by writing down what you weigh now. Next, write down what you want to weigh. Do this now.

Set a Reachable, Reasonable Goal

Be realistic. Losing 10 pounds (4.5 kg) is a lot easier to deal with than losing 50 pounds (22.7 kg). Make a list of all the reasons you want to lose weight and keep it with you or post it in several visible places such as the bathroom mirror, your desk, and your windshield. This is also a good time to make a list of any reasons why you want to continue to be overweight, if any. Go deep.

Don't Buy Into False Images

Trimming the fat from our bodies should not only be for the sake of vanity, but for optimum health. Select what is ideal for your body and don't be overly influenced by unhealthy images that fashion magazines, commercials, TV shows, and movies promote. Remember to recognize what a real person's body looks like. You know what looks right for you.

Why Are You Really Overweight?

It may help to explore the emotional causes and stress that may be at the core of your weight gain. Many of us unconsciously need to physically insulate ourselves out of emotional protection because of past hurts, sexual violation, and fear of intimacy. Weight gain can have its roots in many psychological causes, including stress, emotional insecurity, and depression.

If this sounds like you, consider seeing a therapist who specializes in food issues. Prayer, meditation, guided visualization, and yoga can all help to provide serenity and stability in your life. It can also help to write about your feelings and why you may use food as a drug. Affirm daily, "I will only put health-giving, vital foods into my body."

Clear Out Food Clutter

The first step in learning to eat for optimal weight is to clear out food clutter. Clean out the cupboards and give away, compost, or throw out all the foods containing undesirable ingredients such as sugar, hydrogenated oil, and artificial flavors, and coloring. This way you make room for healthy choices.

Getting rid of unnecessary stuff in your life will help you let go of weight as well. You are making change happen! Make some charity happy or have a yard sale and let this be a metaphor for getting lighter in your life.

Start a piggy bank and save daily what you would spend on a soda, latte, or candy bar. Use the money to buy new clothes, CDs, or donate to a food bank.

Create a Healthy Shopping List

Before you go shopping create a weekly shopping list, and do your best to stick with it. Read the labels you need to and avoid aisles that aren't relevant to your new healthy diet. If you buy fresh fruits, vegetables, nuts, and seeds, they won't even have ingredient labels. You won't need to go down the cereal, cookie, bread, frozen food, and candy aisles. You'll find that food shopping can get done a lot quicker and cost less. *Remember, you don't need to stop eating, only improve what you eat!*

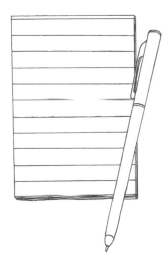

Skip This!

You'll be surprised how frequently sugar (of many different varieties like high fructose corn syrup, sucrose, and dextrose) is listed. Cutting back gradually can be an intelligent place to start so you don't shock your system. Banish sugar from your home. You'll find lots of helpful information about dealing with your sugar addiction in the book *Beat Sugar Addiction Now!* by Jacob Teitelbaum, M.D., and Chrystle Fiedler and in the section "Curbing Cravings" in this chapter.

Start the Day the Right Way

One of the healthiest ways to start your day—and break the fast from the night before—is with a cup of room-temperature water to which the juice of half a fresh lemon has been added. This beverage is naturally diuretic, and the slightly sour taste will improve liver function, aid fat metabolism, and promote good bowel health. If you can, drink six or more glasses of water in the morning.

Best Foods for Weight Loss

Beneficial foods for weight loss include apples, beets, broccoli, carrots, celery, citrus fruits, collards, cranberries, grapefruit, green leafy vegetables, papaya, parsley, unpasteurized sauerkraut, sea vegetables, and raw sunflower and pumpkin seeds. Consume fruit instead of fruit juices to get the benefit of the fiber. Try having a piece of fruit for dessert instead of a sugary treat; however, eat a wide range of foods and know that too much fruit can add too much sugar, though natural, to one's regime.

Write It Down

Keep a food journal of what you eat and drink for a week to gain insight about what your diet really looks like. If you do eat something that's not part of your plan, rather than feel guilty, observe and write about what emotional factors were driving you. Were you tired, bored, or anxious? How did you feel after eating it? If the food you eat has no nutritional value, it really isn't worth consuming. Don't even have junk food in the house!

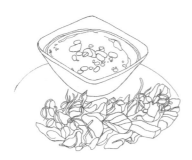

Fill Up on Soup and Salad

It helps to begin a meal with a bowl of soup or a salad to satisfy hunger. You'll use less salad dressing if you toss it in a bowl rather than pouring it on a salad. Make your own salad dressing with extra-virgin olive oil. Most other oils get heated to a temperature over 200°F (93°C) when being pressed, which makes them produce free radicals.

The Subject of Snacking

If you feel tired, try taking a nap or walk as a no-calorie way to get energized rather than having a snack. Have a cup of herbal tea for a snack with a sliced apple.

Eating in the Evening

Right after dinner, floss and brush your teeth to discourage any more food consumption. If you must eat something, choose an apple or raw carrot. Keeping one's room a bit chillier at night uses more calories and also keeps your skin from getting dried out.

Eating on the Go

People often fall off their diets because they are out and about and have no healthy foods with them. Get yourself a cute lunch box and you'll be inspired to always have an assortment of raw and healthy foods with you.

Meal Shifting

You may want to consider having lunch rather than dinner as the main meal. That's because you require fuel more at midday than at night. Some people only need to eat two meals a day. Consider how you may shift meals if at all possible, even if it is just on weekends or holidays. Even worse than eating a big dinner is snacking into the night.

Curbing Cravings

When you change your diet, it's natural to crave what you're missing. Usually the most difficult withdrawal time is the first two months. Rotate the colors of foods you eat to diminish cravings. Drink green drinks to discourage cravings, because they are very alkalinizing.

To gain more control, start by writing down what tempts you. This will make it easier to avoid it. Remember, the food that you crave most, such as potato chips, coffee, or chocolate, is very likely the thing that challenges your health the most. Here are some remedies for specific cravings.

If you have PMS cravings: Eat avocados.

If you crave salt: A craving for salty foods like chips may indicate that minerals are needed. Wanting potato chips and salty, crunchy foods may also indicate anger and frustration.

Include mineral-rich sea vegetables like kelp, dulse, or hiziki in your diet. Their natural iodine content nourishes the thyroid gland, which governs metabolism, thus improving the rate at which digestion functions. Sea vegetables can be added to many dishes and will reduce the amount of salt used to flavor food. They are also available in tablet or capsule form.

Commercial salts are often heated to 1,400°F (760°C), have their minerals removed, and then are sold to the vitamin companies. That's why just one chip never satisfies! Instead, try Celtic salt, which is unrefined and naturally rich in trace minerals.

Support for Overeaters

Overeating can be due to the body's incessant quest for nutritional satisfaction that it never receives from processed foods. Overeaters also eat for comfort when stressed, anxious, or depressed. If you are having trouble controlling how much you eat, consider tapping the group power of Overeaters Anonymous, which features the twelve steps that are used in Alcoholics Anonymous. You can attend meetings in person, online, and over the phone that can give you the support you need to overcome the compulsion to eat beyond the need for nutrition. Visit www.oa.org.

If you crave sweets: Craving sweets is often an attempt to elevate the mood. It may also indicate that the body needs more fluids, minerals, or protein. Incorporate more protein sources such as raw nuts, sun-cured olives, or spirulina in your diet. Include some sweet, satisfying, and nourishing foods like winter squashes, carrots, Jerusalem artichokes, parsnips, sweet potatoes, and fresh fruit rather than refined sugars and carbohydrates. Eating celery also diminishes sweet food cravings.

Slow down and savor the natural sweetness in food, noticing it's "full," containing nutrients, rather than "hollow," empty of nutrients. Get into enjoying herb teas without sweeteners. Or use natural sweeteners such as stevia.

A dose of bitter herbal tincture (available at natural product stores, usually made from bitter herbs such as gentian) can help dispel a sweet craving.

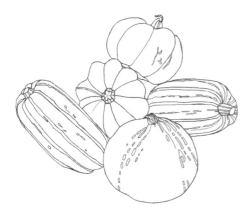

The Problem with Sugar

Remember, even though sugar can give you a quick burst of energy, that buzz is quickly gone, leaving you more tired than you were to begin with and craving more sugar. Eating excess sweets can also cause excess urination, tooth sensitivity, constipation, mouth sores, and grogginess. Chemical sweeteners can actually cause you to crave more sweets by upsetting blood sugar levels.

Try This!

When you feel a sugar urge coming on, visualize breathing in deeply the color pink to warm the heart with its healing ray. Wearing rose quartz can help connect you to this pink light.

The Benefits of Being Sugar Free

Eating less sugar, and better yet, cutting it out of your diet, can only improve your physical and emotional health. Check out one of my earlier books, *Addiction-Free Naturally*. It is all about getting free from sugar, food additions, caffeine, alcohol, and other substances with the help of food, herbs, supplements, flower essences, and essential oils.

How I Gave Up Chocolate

I was able to give up eating chocolate by stuffing a date with raw almond butter; the combination of sweet and fat is very satisfying. Not all fats are negative. Weight gain is more related to refined carbohydrates that stimulate insulin production and therefore fat storage.

Good to Know!

In recent years there has been a lot of attention on reducing carbohydrates to lose weight. There is a big difference between the refined carbohydrates in a muffin or bagel and the carbs in an apple or carrot. Get your carbs from fresh fruit and vegetables rather than processed foods.

If you crave fats: Fat is not a flavor, but a carrier of flavor. We need good-quality fats for energy and warmth and to protect our nerves and keep our organs in their right place. Consuming a daily tablespoon of hemp seed oil or using more raw, healthful fats like raw-soaked nuts, avocados, and sun-cured olives gives the body beneficial essential fatty acids that can help emulsify fat. If you crave avocados and nuts, eat them, but balance them with lots of greens, celery, and cucumbers.

If you crave caffeine: When craving stimulants, which may indicate feeling dull or depressed, play upbeat music or drink some ginger or peppermint tea. Drink cardamom tea or smell cardamom or jasmine essential oil.

Handling Cravings in the Moment

Cravings are more likely to occur when you are hungry or experiencing low blood sugar. Most cravings will pass within a few minutes. Taking a few deep, slow breaths may help. If there is a food you crave, save the wrapper even after the food is gone and just breathe in the aroma.

Distract Yourself

If you really want a specific food, try putting a wedge between you and the craving. Do something else. Take a walk, call a friend, read a good book. If you are still craving it, eat it and observe how you feel.

It's best to not eat between meals, but if you really need a snack, try:

- Celery sticks
- Nuts
- Flax crackers
- Sun-cured olives
- An alkalinizing green juice such as celery, cucumber, parsley, apple juice diluted with water, or a few blades of wheatgrass

Avoid Drinking Your Calories

For the most part, it's best to eat your calories. Not only is it more satisfying to chew but drinking soda, or even healthy fruit juices can quickly elevate blood sugar levels. If you are going to drink your calories, choose freshly pressed juices because bottled juices are pasteurized and lack enzymes. Also, choose juices that contain fiber to slow the absorption of any sugars that may be present. Because even many fresh-pressed juices are very sweet, consider diluting them with at least 50 percent water before consuming.

Healing Food Allergies to Reach Your Optimal Weight

Eating foods that you are allergic to can make weight loss just about impossible, because they can cause bloating and be difficult to digest. Very often the foods we crave are the ones we are allergic to. Common allergens include wheat, dairy, eggs, corn, sugar, yeast, citrus, peanuts, chocolate, coffee, soy, potatoes, tomatoes, fish, and shellfish.

How Allergies Affect Your Body

When an allergen is consumed, the body gets stressed and produces adrenaline, which increases the heart rate, causes the liver to move glucose, and enlarges pupils. This can actually cause you to feel temporarily comforted, because the immune system is working overtime. A sign of food allergy is when your weight fluctuates by several pounds a day. Allergy-triggered fluid retention may be the cause.

Some people with eating disorders may actually have food intolerances that can cause damage to the intestinal lining when the food is consumed. This makes food abusers more likely to choose foods that require little digestion, such as sugar, white flour products, and alcohol.

Do-It-Yourself Allergy Test

Having an allergy test may be a good idea, because we often crave the foods we are sensitive to in order to avoid withdrawal. You can do the Coca Pulse Test yourself to see whether you have a food allergy. First, check your pulse on an empty stomach for six seconds and then multiply by ten to get your pulse by the minute. Then thirty to sixty minutes after a meal containing a suspected allergen, check your pulse again. If it is faster than it was previously, that can be a sign that you are having a reaction to a food that was consumed.

The Practice of Kinesiology

Kinesiology can be another method for determining a food allergy. But you'll need to see a practitioner. He or she will have you stand with your dominant arm, usually right, extended out to your side. The practitioner will then push down on the extended arm, as you hold a small amount of a suspected food either in your mouth or in front of your stomach. If you can easily hold your arm up and out while someone pushes down on it, you're most likely tolerant of the food being tested. If you become weak and unable to resist, that can be a sign that you are allergic to the substance being tested.

The Value of a Raw-Foods Diet in Weight Loss

A raw-foods diet enables you to eat delicious food and maintain your body's optimal weight. You'll also have more energy, so it will be easier to exercise.

Personally, I had been trying to lose 10 pounds (4.5 kg) for years and never really did. Adopting a raw-foods diet enabled me to get to my desired weight effortlessly and with great vitality and the best health ever. Please check out my book *Rawsome!* It is filled with delicious, healthful, and easy-to-prepare recipes.

Before You Begin a Raw Diet

Take a "before raw" photo of yourself. Take one after six months of raw. Write about your health history. Keep a food journal and write down goals in the present tense. Write down five limiting beliefs and replace them with affirmations. For example, "I am fat" can be replaced with "Every day I am making healthier choices." Make a list of five foods you would be better off giving up.

Eating Raw 101

An easy way to begin to experience the benefits of raw food is to start each meal with something raw. Or make one meal a day raw. Have salad as the main dish rather than a side.

Gradually increase the proportion of raw food and decrease the amount of cooked food. Try a new fruit or vegetable every week.

Have baked or steamed rather than fried foods. Let go of prepackaged foods, instant fixes, frozen meals, and ready-to-eat, chemically tainted, and refined empty foods that damage health.

If you overdo sugars, eat greens and healthy fats to balance. Buy groceries at natural food stores or markets that sell organic produce, and avoid regular grocery stores. Select foods that are organic and in season as much as possible.

Eating Raw on the Go

Americans consume 65 percent of their meals outside the home. But if you're concerned about eating healthy food, you're more likely to eat at home, where you can ensure quality control. Sometimes, though, you'll need to eat out. That's okay; eating healthfully away from home is easier than ever before.

Raw and healthful restaurants are a growing trend, and if there's one in your area, you're in luck. However, maybe your friends want to eat elsewhere, or there are no raw-food restaurants in your area. Don't worry; you can always eat a salad and make it superhealthy.

If the restaurant doesn't have a salad bar, examine a salad off the menu, being sure to check the list of ingredients carefully and ask the waitstaff to omit items such as cheese and croutons. Consider having a salad as an appetizer or another kind as an entrée. Instead of having the proverbial chicken or fish with rice, potatoes, or pasta, if you do eat animal foods, have fish or chicken on a salad. If a salad doesn't seem filling enough, bring a ripe avocado with you to the restaurant and discreetly add it to your salad for a more complete meal. For salad dressing, ask for olive oil and lemon juice. Or you can bring your own raw dressing from home.

For breakfast, ask for a fresh fruit platter. Tell the waitperson you want more fruit instead of cottage cheese. No fruit platter? Perhaps they have a ripe melon.

Good to Know!

If you go raw, you'll lose weight, and it's possible that it will be dramatic enough to concern your family and friends. Though this may happen initially, usually you'll gain back some weight, though of better quality. If you have any questions, see your health care practitioner for advice.

Do your best, but be prepared to compromise, and be gracious with the waitstaff. Thank them for answering your questions and procuring your special requests.

Eating Raw When Entertaining

When you are invited to a dinner party, inform your host of your food program as soon as you receive the invitation, but tell him or her not to fret or go to any trouble to accommodate you. Offer instead to bring to the party a raw dish that you can eat as a main course and that others can try, if they wish, as a side dish.

When you're talking to your host or friends, avoid preaching the benefits of the raw diet. Once you've told them that you're on a raw diet, they may ask about it, but if they do not, don't force the details on them.

Introduce Your Guests to the Value of Eating Raw

When you are the host of a dinner party, you can introduce your guests to the delights of a raw diet without any lecturing at all, simply by offering a wide range of delicious raw foods.

Presentation of food is highly important, and perhaps even more so with raw foods. It's always best to prepare dishes as close as possible to the time of consumption so that the fresh foods won't wilt or discolor. Serve foods on beds of color: greens, grated carrots, or sliced cabbage. Use garnishes that complement the dish in both flavor and color. Serve your food on beautiful plates, bowls, and platters.

Going raw will lower the cost of traveling, because raw foods are generally less expensive than cooked ones. In fact, you can even plan your vacation around your diet. Travel to a fruit-filled tropical paradise during mango or durian season. Visit the wilds of Maine during blueberry season. Enjoy the hospitality of the South during peach or orange season.

When traveling by car, bring an ice chest and carry in it raw salad dressings. During hot weather, keep your fruits and vegetables in the chest, too. A cutting board, knife, sprout bag, bowls, and utensils are also useful.

Prepare dried fruits and vegetables before a trip. Take flax crackers, raw granola, sunflower and pumpkin seeds, and sun-cured olives. Keep with you a small container of unpasteurized miso; it can be stirred into a bit of purified water to make a soup broth.

Travel with superfoods such as powders or tablets of barley grass, wheatgrass, spirulina, or blue-green algae for the nutrients and energy they provide, especially if you can't count on finding fresh vegetables.

Make it part of the adventure to find health food stores and restaurants that serve salads. Stop at roadside markets. Take the opportunity to eat simply. Have an adventure!

Make Mealtimes Peaceful

Whether you change your diet a little or a lot, or even go raw, and whether you eat out or at home, make the time you spend eating peaceful. Too often mealtime is a rush and continuation of the stress in our daily lives.

Before eating, always serve yourself, rather than eating out of containers. Serve portions to people at the table and avoid country-style platters on the table.

Sit down, relax, look at your food, and visualize it nourishing you. Say a blessing or take a few deep breaths to get calm and centered.

Focus on Your Food

When eating, it is important to be focused. Avoid eating while reading, driving, or watching TV. When I was at my heaviest, I could eat three bowls of cereal at breakfast, simply because I kept unconsciously eating while reading the newspaper and never felt truly nourished.

Eat Slow: Take It Bite by Bite

As you eat, put your fork down between bites. Chew your food better, on both sides to encourage facial symmetry. It takes about twenty minutes for your brain to receive the message that you are satisfied. You may find that using a smaller plate and a cocktail fork or chopsticks to dine reminds you to appreciate each bite. It is okay to leave some food on your plate.

Eat as a family or with friends if you can. But keep in mind that if you talk too much during a meal, you may remain unappreciative of the food you eat. However, some conversations during meals will beneficially slow down eating.

 Cure Caution:

Using herbs for weight loss in therapeutic dosages during pregnancy is not recommended.

 Healing Herbs for Weight Loss

A multitude of herbs have been used to help weight loss. The easiest way to start using them is to spice up your meals with flavorful culinary herbs, such as cayenne, cinnamon, coriander, garlic, and ginger. These herbs are warming, strengthen the spleen, improve circulation, and encourage metabolism and the burning of brown fat and are thus referred to as *thermogenic* or *metabolism increasing*.

These herbs can help you lose weight by providing important nutrients, improving digestion, and curbing cravings. Start with one and add more as needed. If you have a medical condition, talk to your health practitioner before taking any herb for weight loss.

Burdock is a chologogue, choleretic, diuretic, expectorant, laxative (mild), nutritive, and rejuvenative. Burdock improves the elimination of metabolic wastes through the liver, lymph nodes, large intestines, lungs, kidneys, and skin. It makes an excellent spring detox or fasting tea. It also contains vitamin C, calcium, iron, magnesium, potassium, and zinc and a starch called inulin, which aids in the metabolism of carbohydrates. It can be used as a tea or tincture or eaten as a vegetable. I like to grate it into salads. Burdock stimulates bile production, thus enabling fat breakdown in the body.

Cayenne is high in beta-carotene and vitamin C. It causes the brain to secrete more endorphins. It is considered thermogenic, meaning it can rev up metabolism and aid in weight loss.

Chickweed has laxative, liver-cleansing, and nutritive properties. Chickweed nourishes the yin fluids and dissolves plaque in the blood vessels and fatty deposits in the body. It reduces inflammation and clears toxins. Chickweed can be added to juices, salad, soup, and other dishes. It contains vitamin C, phosphorus, calcium, copper, zinc, and lecithin.

Cinnamon, a circulatory stimulant and diuretic, contains calcium, iron, magnesium, and zinc. It helps dry dampness in the body and it is also thermogenic.

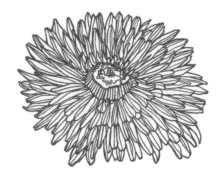

Cola nut is valued as a diuretic and stimulant. Cola nut is used to remedy fatigue and obesity. It does contain caffeine and theobromine. African natives chew the seeds to curb hunger, allay thirst, and enable them to work hard in hot conditions. **Note:** Those with high blood pressure, heart palpitations, and peptic ulcers should avoid this herb because of the caffeine content.

Dandelion leaves and roots are laxative, lithotriptic, and nutritive. Dandelion is also a blood purifier, which aids in the process of filtering and straining wastes from the bloodstream. It is useful in treating obstructions of the gallbladder, liver, pancreas, and spleen. Dandelion is used to help clear the body of old emotions such as anger and fear that can be stored in the liver and kidneys. It is an excellent herb for weight loss, as the root improves fat metabolism and the leaves are diuretic.

Fennel seed was consumed by ancient Greek Olympic athletes so they would gain strength but not weight. Roman women ate fennel seed to prevent weight gain. The poor ate the seeds during the Middle Ages when they had nothing else or during long church sermons or days of fasting to stave off hunger.

Fennel seeds are delightfully sweet and help to curb the appetite by stabilizing blood sugar levels. Fennel is used to improve bloated stomach conditions. Chewing the seeds after a meal freshens the breath.

Flaxseed is rich in omega-3 fatty acids, protein, and vitamins A and B. It contains more vitamin E per volume than any other known seed.

Flaxseeds curb hunger because of their bulk and promote better bowel movements through their colon-lubricating activity. Eat 1 to 2 tablespoons (8 to 16 g) of seeds, chew well, or grind or soak the seeds beforehand. Be sure to consume plenty of fluids to aid this excellent bulk laxative. Better yet, learn to make flaxseed crackers.

Garcinia (*Garcinia cambogia*) is a member of the Clusiaceae family. The rind of the fruit is thermogenic and has been used to treat obesity by helping to curb hunger by making meals more filling.

This plant prevents the body from turning carbohydrates into fat by inhibiting the synthesis of fatty acids. It lowers the production of low-density lipoproteins and increases the production of glycogen. It contains hydroxycitric acid, similar to the citric acid found in oranges and grapefruits, which reduces appetite, stabilizes blood sugar levels, and enhances digestion. Garcinia also appears to improve the body's ability to burn calories.

Cure Caution:

Guar can cause obstructions in the esophagus and intestines as well as gas and bloating, so it's important to drink plenty of water. Guar gum can also decrease the need for insulin if you are a diabetic. Inform your doctor if you are using it, so that your need for insulin can be decreased if necessary.

Those allergic to citric acid (citrus fruits, tomatoes) may have sensitivities to garcinia, though it has been safely used as a food for many centuries. Avoid it during pregnancy and nursing. Take three capsules one half hour to an hour before each meal.

Ginger rhizomes are choleretic, thermogenic, and improve spleen function. Ginger stimulates amylase concentration in the saliva and aids in the digestion of starches and fatty foods. Ginger is composed of sulfur, protein, and the proteolytic enzyme zingibain.

Guar gum (*Cyamoposis tetragonoloba, C. psoraliodes*) is a member of the Fabaceae (bean) family. The seeds and pods are laxative. Guar gum helps lower serum cholesterol levels and blood glucose levels. It slows down the absorption of carbohydrates. It tends to swell up in the digestive tract, causing a feeling of fullness and thus decreasing hunger. It is used in capsules. Use only the suggested dose.

Gymnema, also known as gurmar (*Gymnema sylvestre*), is a member of the Asclepiadeceae (milkweed) family. Gymnema has long been used to treat obesity.

Gurmar means "sugar destroyer," and when you chew some of this leaf and then place sugar on the tongue, the sweet taste is eliminated in a few seconds. The molecules of the gymnemic acid fill the receptor sites for one to two hours, preventing taste buds from being activated by the sugar molecules in food, and actually block sugar from being absorbed during digestion. Gurmar improves glucose utilization, enhances insulin production, and helps you overcome sugar addiction. It contains stigmasterol, betaine, and choline. **Note:** If you are using gymnema and are insulin dependent, consult with your physician, as insulin medication may need to be readjusted.

Hoodia (*Hoodia gordonii*) looks like a cactus, but it's actually a succulent in the Asclepiadaceous (milkweed) family from the Kalahari Desert in southern Africa. Bushmen from the area have used hoodia for centuries to help ward off hunger during long trips in the desert. That's because hoodia tricks the brain into thinking you've eaten and makes you feel full.

Studies show that it reduces interest in food, delays the time after eating before hunger sets in again, and promotes a full feeling more quickly. It contains a substance known as P57 that is believed to suppress the appetite by affecting the nerve cells that send the brain glucose, causing you to feel satisfied. It is not a stimulant and has no known side effects.

Yerba maté leaves are alterative, antioxidant, antiscorbutic, aperient, astringent, diuretic, rejuvenative, stimulant, stomachic, and tonic. Maté cleanses the blood, stimulates the mind, and respiratory and nervous systems, and decreases the appetite.

Yerba maté contains beta-carotene, vitamins B and C, calcium, iron, magnesium, manganese, potassium, silicon, sulfur, and tannins. The tannin content tends to bind with the caffeine, thereby reducing both compounds' effects. Most people who find caffeine impairs sleep will not experience this with maté. **Note:** It's best to avoid consuming maté with meals, as the high tannin content can impair nutrient assimilation. Use cautiously when suffering from anxiety, heart palpitations, and insomnia.

Nettle leaves are used medicinally as an adrenal tonic, alterative, antioxidant, cholagogue, circulatory stimulant, diuretic, endocrine tonic (seed), expectorant, nutritive, rejuvenative (seed), and thyroid tonic (seed). Nettles are used to improve acne, cellulite, and obesity. Nettle leaf and root tone and firm tissue, muscles, arteries, and skin. Nettles help curb the appetite and cleanse toxins from the body.

Because nettles are energizing, they help with motivation to stay on a healthy diet. Nettles contain protein, beta-carotene, xanthophylls, vitamins B, C, E, and K, flavonoids, calcium, chromium, and iron.

Psyllium (*Plantago psyllium, P. ovata*) is a member of the Plantaginaceae (plantain) family. The seeds and outer husk of seeds are employed as a laxative and stool softener and are traditionally used to treat constipation and obesity. One teaspoon is taken in a bit of water or juice to curb hunger by causing a feeling of fullness in the stomach and promotes normal elimination. Drink it quickly before it jells up. It can also be taken in capsules.

Psyllium is high in mucilage and essential fatty acids. The seeds absorb eight to fourteen times their weight in water. Their fibrous qualities make them laxative, yet they also provide intestinal bulk, which can stop diarrhea. Because they tend to swell and create a feeling of fullness, they can help curb the appetite.

Note: Always use psyllium with plenty of liquids—otherwise it can cause constipation. Psyllium can dilute digestive enzymes and is best taken between meals—especially before bed or first thing upon rising rather than with food.

Green tea contains carotenoids, chlorophyll, caffeine, theophylline, theobromine, gamma-amino butyric acid, polysaccharides, fats, vitamins C and E, manganese, potassium, zinc, and fluoride. Green tea is diuretic and thermogenic.

Green tea prevents the blood from "clumping together" and forming clots that can lead to stroke. The catechin content of green tea helps to break down cholesterol and increase its elimination through the bowels.

Green tea also helps to keep blood sugar levels moderate and promotes clarity and energy. Even though caffeine gets a bad rap, the caffeine in green tea increases the synthesis of catecholamines, which are stimulant chemicals that relay nerve impulses in the brain.

Green tea has about 25 mg of caffeine per cup (black tea has about 35 to 40). The caffeine content of green tea is about as much as a soda and one-third to half as much as a cup of coffee. **Note:** Excessive use of green tea can cause nervous irritability and aggravate ulcers. Avoid it in cases of hypertension and insomnia.

Health food stores carry herbal combinations in tea, capsule, and tablet form that can be used along with a good diet and exercise program to help you let go of unnecessary weight.

Weight Balance Vitamins and Mineral Therapy

As the body burns fats, it produces metabolic waste products known as ketones and lipid peroxides. Using an antioxidant vitamin can help keep the body healthy during this process. B complex, vitamin C, zinc, and calcium-magnesium can decrease sugar cravings.

Taking 200 micrograms of **GTF (glucose tolerance factor)** chromium can be very effective in keeping blood sugar levels stable, helps insulin work more efficiently, and keeps your mind off sweets. Chromium also has been found to decrease blood lipid levels. A maximum of five tablets can be taken throughout the day, if needed. Decrease this as you need it less because of your improved diet.

L-glutamine can help satisfy the body's craving for sugar and refined carbohydrates. The amino acid L-glycine also helps you control sugar addiction. Both amino acids have a calming effect upon the brain. L-phenylalanine also helps the brain feel satisfied. Both phenylalanine and tyrosine are thermogenic.

A daily supplement of **fish or krill oil** that contains omega-3 essential fatty acids can actually help improve the body's metabolism of fat and reduce fat cravings.

Lipoic acid helps protect the liver against toxins and is an antioxidant. **Coenzyme Q$_{10}$** (also known as ubiquinone) is an antioxidant that improves the ability to metabolize fats. It is present in almost all cells and also tends to decline with age.

Holistic Therapies and Practices
Aromatherapy

Instead of eating sweets, smell the sweet aromas of anise, fennel, and spearmint essential oils to pleasure the brain and dispel unnecessary urges to eat. Here are other ways aromatherapy can help you meet your weight loss goals:

- Bitter orange also helps deter a desire for sweets.
- Essential oils that are good to use for massage when you want to lose weight include cypress, juniper, and rosemary.
- Grapefruit essential oil helps those who eat when under pressure. Bergamot essential oil helps deter food addictions.
- The flower essence cherry plum, one of the Bach Flower Remedies, is useful if you tend to go on eating binges.

Try Acupressure

If you're feeling hungry between meals, try acupressure. A valuable pressure point to use to curb hunger is located in the indentation in the face in front of each ear.

Be Nice to Yourself

If you are kind to yourself, you have a much better chance at making it to your ideal weight and maintaining it. That's because negative self-talk and blame can trigger overeating. It's important to find ways other than food to nourish yourself.

Consider the sensual delights of a warm bubble bath, a massage, reading a great novel, or walking in a beautiful environment, whether it be in nature or a fabulous art museum. Take a walk after a meal rather than having dessert. Take up a craft. Rather than keeping your hands in the chip bowl while watching a movie or hanging out with friends, learn to create something beautiful or practical.

I love to embroider designs on T-shirts for my grandchildren, knit baby blankets, sew doll clothes, and do bead work. Find something that suits you.

Make a list of all the alternative ways to bring nurturing enjoyment into life, besides food, and start doing them. Do this right now.

Connect with Your Inner Self

Place a mirror on the refrigerator as a traditional feng shui remedy to deter overeating. Make eye contact in the mirror before opening the fridge to feel more connected to who you really are. In addition, put a photo of yourself at your slimmest (preferably in a bathing suit) on the refrigerator.

Avoid Temptation

If you can't have certain foods at home like sugar, white bread, or white rice, don't buy them. Use the front door to enter your house rather than enter through the kitchen, or food will be the first thing you think of. Place a table between the fridge and where you sit in the living room to psychologically block food cravings. Avoid walking by the vending machine or other places of temptation at work.

If You Wish to Gain Weight

If you're underweight, gaining a few pounds can help ground you so you achieve a healthier balance. Foods that can help you gain weight include avocados, bananas, dried fruits, pumpkin seeds, sunflower seeds, and nut butters. Have this easy-to-make smoothie one or two times a day, including some of these foods along with regular meals.

Weight Gain Smoothie

2 cups (570 ml) raw almond milk
1½ ripe bananas
3 pitted dates, soaked 20 minutes
1 tablespoon (15 g) raw tahini

Blend. Enjoy once or twice daily.

Eating Well for Optimal Health

Whether your goal is to lose or gain weight, the process can teach you how to eat for optimal wellness, to be good to yourself and take advantage of the wide variety of natural remedies that are available. It can also help you add years of joy and happiness to your life. May your journey reveal your most beautiful self ever!

If You Have Anorexia or Bulimia

Both anorexia and bulimia are more likely to occur in women (about 90 percent), but do occur in men. Cultural images promoted in the media of extremely thin models can give young people false and distorted ideas of body image, and what "real" people actually look like, and contribute to these eating disorders.

The Three Steps to Healing

These three steps can help you begin to heal from anorexia and/or bulimia:

1. Correct any underlying health problem (such as low thyroid or biochemical imbalance) that you might have.

2. Establish healthy eating habits and regain enough weight to be out of danger of physical impairment.

3. Get counseling by a professional trained in eating disorders to help resolve conflicts about growing up, sexuality, parental and sibling strife, control, denying the self and life, as well as depression.

What Is Anorexia?

The word *anorexia* is Greek for "without a longing to eat." Anorexia nervosa is chronic undereating, obsession with thinness, and a fear of weight gain. Anorexia can be diagnosed when weight loss leads to a body weight 85 percent of that considered normal.

Anorexia can lead to amenorrhea in women, anemia, hair loss, constipation, low blood pressure, edema, sleep disturbances, nutritional deficiency, hypothermia, hypoglycemia, hirsutism, osteoporosis later in life, cardiac episodes, emaciation, and a lifetime of digestive disorders.

When to See Your M.D.

Both anorexia and bulimia are serious conditions and can be life threatening, so it's important to work with a trusted health practitioner to help you get well. This information is intended for educational purposes. Check with your holistic doctor to see which of these natural cures may help you.

What Is Bulimia?

The word *bulimia* is from the Greek and means "ox hunger." Bulimia nervosa is a repeated cycle of eating excessively, called bingeing, and then purging, either by vomiting or through the abuse of laxatives. This is usually done secretly.

Vomiting and laxatives are not an effective way to lose weight, as most bingeing is done with refined carbohydrates, which are very quickly absorbed and can have devastating effects upon the teeth, stomach, and esophagus. People have died from both anorexia and bulimia.

Anorexia and bulimia are classified as separate psychiatric disorders, but sometimes they over-lap. The hormonelike substance cholecystokinin (CCK), which signals the brain that the stomach is full, does not kick in for those with bulimia until they regain normal eating habits. Bingeing can also be aggravated by neurotransmitters that have gone haywire due to a diet that causes the body to demand instant sweets and refined carbohydrates.

Both conditions are eating disorders that result, in part, from having abnormally low endorphin levels, the feel-good hormone. Fasting, binge-ing, purging, excessive dieting, starving oneself, and overexercising all elevate endorphin levels temporarily, which can make it very difficult for people with these disorders to change.

Many anorexics are perfectionists, and eating disorders often affect the good student who seemingly has no problems.

Good to Know!

In families, it is important to give well-behaved children as much attention as the ones who may have problems.

How Food Intolerances Affect Eating Disorders

If you have an eating disorder, you may actually have food intolerances such as to gluten, which, when consumed, can cause damage to the intestinal lining. This makes food abusers more likely to choose foods that require little diges-tion, such as sugar, white flour products, and alcohol. Keep in mind that you are also more likely to binge on foods you are allergic to, such as gluten, dairy, and corn.

Yeast overgrowth, also known as candida, can also be a contributing factor in eating disorders. This can cause people who eat carbohydrates to feel bloated and fat when they consume them.

Write It Down

Keep a daily food journal to observe mood patterns and which foods are binge triggers and to promote awareness.

Improve Appetite Naturally

Taking a dose of digestive bitters, which often contain herbs like centaury, gentian, and orange peel, ten minutes before a meal can increase appetite and aid digestion.

Necessary Nutrients

Eating a high-raw, fresh fruit and vegetable diet that is low in calories and health giving can help you reach a healthy weight if you have an eating disorder. Increase food levels gradually as you heal.

It's also important to focus on foods that calm the spirit, nourish the stomach and spleen, and tonify the heart, like pumpkins, winter squash, and yams. Watery cooked black quinoa, millet, or black rice with some vegetables cooked into them are ideal. Use seasonings such as cilantro, cinnamon, garlic, and ginger. Also include some raw juices. Persimmons and ripe pineapple are good fruits to use, rich in enzymes.

Helpful Herbs from A-Z

Herbs are a natural way to help ease the symptoms of anorexia and bulimia and encourage appetite. You can take them as supplements, or in a tea or tincture.

California poppy: Calms the nerves. For anxiety, hyperactivity, insomnia, restlessness, and stress.

Catnip: Helps amenorrhea, anxiety, flatulence, hyperactivity, hysteria, indigestion, nausea, and restlessness.

Chamomile: Helps restore an exhausted nervous system.

Cloves: For anorexia, bulimia, depression, flatulence, indigestion, stomach cramps, and vomiting.

Dandelion: Leaves help anemia. Root improves fat metabolism. Improves liver function.

Eleuthero: For debility and convalescence. Helps depression, fatigue, nervous breakdown, and gives support during stress.

Ginger: Helps amenorrhea, cramps, dyspepsia, flatulence, indigestion, and nausea.

Skip This!

Eliminate caffeine, which can aggravate feelings of anxiety and depression.

Hops: For anorexia, anxiety, indigestion, irritable bowel, and restlessness. Helps you put on weight and assimilate food better. Stimulates digestive secretions. Also calms anxiety and nervousness.

Lemon balm: Helps protect the cerebrum from excessive stimuli. Calms anxiety. Benefits depression, nausea, and nervousness.

Licorice root: Soothes an irritated digestive tract, even one raw from bulimic vomiting. Improves debility, emotional instability, indigestion, and stress.

Marshmallow root: Soothes an irritated digestive tract, even one raw from the effects of bulimic vomiting. Softens harsh emotions such as anger and frustration. Demulcent, laxative, nutritive, rejuvenative, and vulnerary.

Milk thistle seed: Improves liver function and helps stimulate protein synthesis in the liver, thus reversing damage.

Oatstraw: Nutritive and supportive for the nervous system. For debility associated with appetite loss. Helps anxiety, convalescence, depression, exhaustion, and stress.

Passionflower: Quiets the central nervous system. For anxiety, anger, hysteria, nervous breakdown, and stress. Anti-inflammatory, nervine, and sedative.

Peppermint/spearmint: Improves dyspepsia, fatigue, flatulence, indigestion, irritable bowel, nausea, stomachache, and stress.

Poria: Strengthens digestion. Improves anxiety, bloating, convalescence, diarrhea, dyspepsia, and edema.

Saint-John's-wort: Inhibits serotonin breakdown, while enhancing its efficiency. For anxiety, depression, and irritability.

Skullcap: Enhances awareness and calmness. Aids anxiety, emotional trauma, fear, hysteria, restlessness, and stress.

Slippery elm bark: Soothes an irritated, raw digestive tract, helping to rebuild its mucosal lining.

Valerian: For stress and anxiety. Helps hypochondria, nervous breakdown, overeating, and restlessness.

Vervain: Improves nutrient assimilation. Helps relieve agitation, anorexia, anxiety, depression, hysteria, nervousness, and stress.

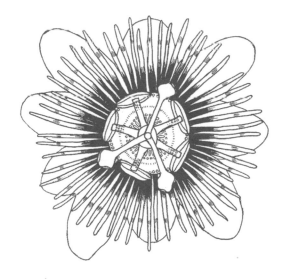

Chinese Remedies

A Chinese patent medicine to consider is **Ren Shen Yang Ying Wan**, which nourishes the heart and spleen and calms the spirit. Another is **Shih Chuan Da Bu Wan (Ten Flavor Tea)**, which tonifies the heart, spleen, and blood. It improves poor appetite and digestion, debility, and anxiety.

Well-Being Supplements

Low levels of **zinc** have been associated with both anorexia and bulimia, so you may want to supplement with this mineral. Studies indicate that zinc in a sulfate form is most effective. The liquid form is easier to absorb and ideal in case of low hydrochloric acid production due to eating disorders. Zinc also improves the senses of smell and taste.

Calcium and **magnesium** are nourishing to the nervous system and can help prevent further bone loss, leading to likeliness of fractures. **Iron** in a chelated form can help correct anemia. **Essential fatty acids** found in a high-quality fish oil and a **B-complex** vitamin help to stabilize the emotional body. Taking **beta-carotene** as a supplement can help heal irritated mucous membranes of the body, irritated from lack of nourishment, vomiting, and laxative use.

Helpful Amino Acids

L-glutamine helps stabilize blood sugar and enhances mental clarity. **Tryptophan** is an essential amino acid needed to make serotonin, which helps balance emotions, aids sleep, and controls pain. The amino acid L-tyrosine can reduce depression and is a precursor to serotonin. **DLPA** (D-phenylalanine) works as an antidepressant. It is used to make adrenaline and tyrosine.

SAM-e can help elevate your mood if you feel depressed by elevating levels of serotonin, dopamine, and phosphatides and improving the ability for neurotransmitters to bind to receptor sites. It's needed for neuronal membrane integrity, neurotransmitter synthesis, and energy metabolism. It also increases the binding of neurotransmitters to receptors and improves the fluidity of brain cell membranes.

Holistic Practices

Homeopathic remedies to consider for eating disorders include:

Aconitum napellus: For fright that causes appetite loss.

Arsenicum album: For exhaustion, vomiting, and fear of poisoning, which is worse after eating.

Cinchona: For eating disorders and associated emotional sensitivity.

Gelsenium: For weakness, dullness, and apathy. Helps with lack of thirst.

Ignatia: For fears of gaining weight and rejection by others.

Natrum muriaticum: Helps ease dry skin and lips, constipation, and fears of rejection.

Phosphoric acid: For apathy toward oneself and food.

Platina: Eases obsessiveness about appearance and egomania.

Sepia: For irritability, indifference, and the desire to be alone. Helps those who disgusted by food and odors, which cause nausea.

Flower Essences

Cerato is for when you lack confidence in your own decisions.

Cherry plum is for when you feel unclean about yourself.

Larch helps those who feel inferior and expect to fail.

Rock water helps those who suppress their inner needs and are hard on themselves.

The flower essence **clematis** is for people who have an aversion to the physical world, including themselves. They follow punishing diets even if they have an adverse effect upon their health. This remedy mellows their attitude and helps them to have a more positive relationship with the world.

Natural Practices to Help You Heal

Practice prayer, meditation, guided visualization, and yoga to enhance serenity and stability in your life. Professional support, nutritional therapy, and the support of family and friends can help you find the road back to health!

Chapter 8

INCREASE ENERGY

Everything is energy and that's all there is to it. Match the frequency of the reality you want and you cannot help but get that reality. It can be no other way. This is not philosophy. This is physics.

—Albert Einstein

Are you tired of being tired? When you make your bed in the morning, do you feel like getting back into it? When you don't have enough energy, everything you need to do is more difficult and can leave you feeling cranky and overwhelmed.

Before you try natural remedies, it's important to rule out any medical reasons for fatigue. Feeling tired can be a sign that you have a condition such as hypothyroidism, in which your thyroid is sluggish, chronic Lyme disease, hypoglycemia, low blood sugar, anemia, a lack of iron in the blood, other nutritional deficiencies, and allergies (both food and environmental). Talk to your health care practitioner about what tests you may need to determine the cause of your fatigue and how to treat it.

Plug into Natural Energy Practices

When you need power in your house, for a lamp, TV, or computer, you put a socket into a plug. It's the same with natural practices that we plug into our lives to boost energy. The first step is deciding which habits you want to adopt, whether it's using herbs, supplements, aromatherapy, exercise, or yoga. The next step is to practice them daily so energy is there when you need it most.

Good to Know!
Targeting Food Allergies

Eating something you are allergic to can make you feel foggy and groggy. But if you keep a food journal, it will help you pinpoint which foods you're allergic to and are making you tired. Dairy products, wheat, gluten, yeast, citrus, and corn are common culprits. You'll be amazed by how much better you feel by eliminating offending foods. I have seen so many people improve their energy levels simply by avoiding a food allergen.

Necessary Nutrients

Try to make lunch the main meal of the day, because you require more energy midday than in the evening. Foods for sustained energy include chia seeds; soaked, rinsed seeds (pumpkin, sesame, sunflower); nuts high in potassium (especially almonds); beans (a rich source of glucose, the body's preferred food); fresh raw vegetables; and fruit. Chia seeds make an energizing breakfast.

Go Green!

Green foods such as collards, kale, spinach, violets, malva, and dandelion and supergreens such as blue-green algae, spirulina, chlorella, barley grass, and wheatgrass are loaded with nutrients such as beta-carotene, iron, protein, and chlorophyll, the wonderful, oxygen-transporting lifeblood of plants. Sea vegetables such as dulse, kelp, and wakame are excellent foods for those with low thyroid function.

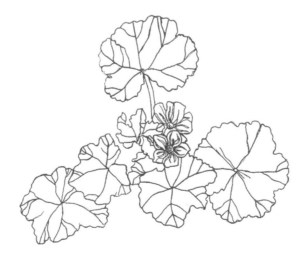

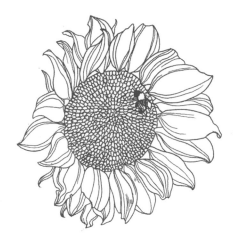

The Buzz on Bee Pollen

Bee pollen can be added to smoothies as an energy booster. If you have pollen allergies, however, start with tiny amounts (one-grain-a-day increments) and increase over a long period of time to 1 teaspoon daily.

Dark Chocolate

If you want a treat, eat dark chocolate. Although it's weaker than caffeine, the chemical theobromine in chocolate is a mild stimulant. Chocolate also contains phenylethylamine, which is a feel-good mood elevator. Choose high-quality, imported dark chocolate with 70 percent or more cocoa content. It has less sugar, and its rich flavor will satisfy you with less. Aim for 1 ounce (2 tablespoons or 28 g) of dark chocolate a few times a week.

The Problem with Sugar and Caffeine

Although sugar and caffeine may give you a quick high, you'll soon crash. That's because when insulin is produced to handle the sugar infusion, your blood sugar drops, leaving you feeling jittery and even more tired. Sugar and caffeine also deplete the body of needed nutrients for energy, such as vitamin B_{12} and calcium. Foods containing heated oils may also make you feel sluggish.

Skip This!

If you can, avoid consuming microwaved food. It's not conducive to building the life energy and vitality you need.

Energizing Drinks

Sipping small amounts of chilled water every thirty minutes sends a signal to your brain to increase alertness and energy. That's because drinking cold water stimulates an adrenaline release by activating the sympathetic or stimulated side of the nervous system, also called the fight-or-flight reaction.

If you've been sitting for too long, your body switches to the parasympathetic nervous system mode, which makes you calm but also can make you feel tired. Cold water will switch you back into the sympathetic, stimulated side of the nervous system and wake you up.

Rehydration will increase your energy quotient too. Keep cold water in the fridge at home and bring it to work in an insulated cup so you can "chill" all day long! Splashing your face with cold water will also increase energy because it, too, stimulates adrenaline to be released.

Green Tea

In addition to water, add green tea to your diet. It does contain some caffeine, but more importantly, it contains L-theanine, an amino acid that has a stress-reducing effect on your brain. It helps to calm you down but leaves your mind clear, sharp, and alert.

Healing Herbs

These herbs have traditionally been used by various cultures to increase stamina. See whether they work for you!

Ashwagandha root benefits lethargy and fatigue, facilitates learning and memory, and is an adaptogen, meaning it helps the body adapt to both physical and emotional stress.

Dandelion root stimulates bile production, thus improving liver function, which when sluggish, can contribute to fatigue. Dandelion root improves digestion and increases vitality.

Ginkgo helps the brain better utilize oxygen, improves mental alertness, and improves peripheral circulation.

Ginseng benefits exhaustion and helps the body deal with stress, adrenal exhaustion, fatigue, immune weakness, and postoperative recovery.

Licorice root is naturally sweet, helps normalize blood sugar levels, and nourishes exhausted adrenal glands.

Schizandra berries improve endurance and are an antioxidant. They improve both fatigue and insomnia.

Well-"B"eing Supplement

A multivitamin mineral complex that includes at least 50 mg of B complex can help cover all the bases to ensure that no deficiencies are contributing to low energy.

Natural Practices

Flower Essences

Flower essences are a gentle way to put more sparkle in your step. The flower essence hornbeam can help those who feel overwhelmed by life. The flower essence olive helps combat fatigue; when you feel you have reached the end of your rope; and when daily activities seem difficult and you wish only to sleep.

Breathing

If your breathing is shallow and your posture poor, your brain may miss out on the recharging properties of oxygen—one of life's free remedies! Tension uses up so much energy, it can leave you feeling wasted. When muscles are tight, circulation is impaired.

When we breathe more fully and deeply, it helps us be more aware, more intuitive, calmer, more alert, more integrated in body, mind, and spirit. Breathing deeply massages the internal organs.

Inhale through the nose to filter out particulates and more directly stimulate the brain. Repressing breathing can repress feelings. There is common lineage in the words *spirit* and *respiration*. Oxygen nourishes every cell in our beings.

Play a musical instrument to increase respiratory capacity. Singing is a great way to increase respiratory capacity. Good posture improves lung capacity.

Breathing Exercises

How we breathe can affect health, beauty, and consciousness. Breathing through the nose warms the air and helps to trap microbes and particles before they reach the lungs. It is better to breathe into the belly rather than only into the chest. When we inhale, it is good to visualize taking in life force and as we exhale, let go of tensions and toxins. Or visualize that you are the ocean and your breathing is the waves. Breathe more deeply and fully and do your best to make the exhale longer than the inhale.

1. **Deep Relaxation Breath:** Lie on the floor with a pillow supporting the knees. Place the palms over the abdomen, with the fingers gently laced just above the navel. Breathe in to a count of three as the abdomen pushes the fingers toward the ceiling. Exhale to a count of five as the fingers and abdomen move toward the floor.

2. **The Complete Breath:** Lie in a quiet place with the arms at the sides, palms facedown. Close the eyes and slowly inhale through the nose as the abdomen expands, then pull the air up into the rib cage and finally the chest. Hold a few seconds. Breathe out slowly while drawing in the abdomen and relaxing the chest and rib cage.

Next, breathe in slowly as in #1, but raise the arms above the head until the backs of the hands touch the floor. Stretch and hold for 10 seconds. As you slowly exhale, bring the arms back to the sides. Repeat the whole procedure several times.

Practice deep breathing exercises daily. Breathe more deeply and slowly into the belly and chest. Inhale deeply for a count of five, allowing the chest and belly to expand. Hold for a count of five (unless you have high blood pressure). Inhale a sniff of air. Exhale slowly to a count of five, relaxing the shoulders and pulling the belly inward. Repeat seven times. Visualize the breath traveling up the spine and down the front of the body. Stand tall with good posture to allow for maximum breathing ability.

Aromatherapy

Essential oils can improve physical and psychological energy levels. Essential oils that boost energy include basil, clary sage, geranium, lavender, lemon, orange, and rosemary. Volatile oils like eucalyptus or spearmint stimulate a part of your brain that triggers alertness.

Peppermint can help wake you up, too. According to a study in the *North American Journal of Psychology*, drivers who were exposed to the scent of peppermint were more alert and had more energy. Chew strong peppermint gum or peppermint mints when driving and during the day to decrease fatigue and increase alertness.

For the other essential oils, place a few drops on a tissue and inhale deeply, or simply take ten deep inhalations from the bottle.

Take More Steps for More Energy

Exercise is important, even when you feel tired. Exercises that are invigorating yet not overtaxing, such as brisk walking, are good places to start. Research at California State University showed that the more steps you take, the more energy you'll have. If you've been sitting, think about how much energy you have at the moment. Next, get up and walk briskly up and down the hall. You'll notice the difference!

When it comes to all types of exercise, though, it's important to avoid overexertion. Exercise is also best done at least two hours before bedtime, so as not to be overstimulating.

Stretch Your Muscles

Gentle yoga and stretches for your neck, shoulders, and back, where most of us hold chronic stress and tension, can also help boost energy. That's because tight muscles are one way we react to real or perceived danger and trigger the fight-or-flight response. When this response becomes chronic, it wears you out, making you feel tired. When you ease the tension in your neck, shoulders, and back, you're signaling your body that it's okay to shut off the fight-or-flight reaction and as a result, you'll have more energy.

When you're at your desk, try twirling a pen or pencil in your fingers, or squeeze a stress ball to release the overall tension in your body. Wiggle your foot or tap your fingers very slowly as you stretch and relax the muscles that are tense.

Visit These Chapters in This Book, Too

Chronic stress and anxiety is guaranteed to make you feel tired. For natural ways to get rid of stress and ease anxiety, visit chapters 2 and 3.

Holistic Therapy: Acupressure

A good do-it-yourself practice to boost energy is acupressure on your outer ear. When you apply pressure to acupressure points all along the outer ear, it helps to clear the head, gets rid of dull pain above the neck, and charges up your entire energy system. Just take your thumb and first finger and go up and down the entire outer ear two or three times and give it a good, brisk rubbing. Rubbing your ears stimulates the energy in your whole body and gets it moving.

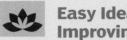 **Easy Ideas for Improving Energy**

1. Reduce exposure to chemicals such as cleaners, art supplies, and pollution.

2. Have water tested and consider getting a water purifier or using bottled water, preferably in glass.

3. Avoid infections by avoiding overexertion, overwork, and junk food.

4. Massage relieves stress and improves circulation and lymphatic drainage.

5. Have regular bed and awakening times. If you take naps, take them at a regular intervals. Try to establish a rhythm.

6. Avoid drinking before bed so you don't need to wake up to urinate. If it helps, add darker curtains to your room. Earplugs may benefit sleep. I love my eye pads!

7. Set a few specific goals for each day and write them down the night before. Consider keeping a journal, which can enhance creativity. Essential oils that enhance creativity include clary sage, helichrysum, neroli, rose, and rosewood.

8. Schedule the most difficult tasks during the time of day when your energy is highest.

9. Put some color into your life. Reds, bright pinks, and orange tones, whether worn or used in décor, help to perk you up. During the day, let the sunshine in!

10. When you have to accomplish tasks, playing some upbeat music can be motivating.

11. After showering, end briefly with cold water to strengthen the nervous system. Several times a day, try spraying your face with cool water that has been lightly scented with pure peppermint oil (use 20 drops essential oil to 8 ounces [1 cup or 235 ml] water).

12. Keep your brain stimulated by using downtime to read uplifting literature more than watching TV. "TV is for the reading impaired" (Terence McKenna).

13. If you are troubled, getting your problems out of your mind and onto a piece of paper makes you feel lighter. Brainstorm possible solutions. Have someone supportive to talk to.

14. Pray, meditate, and keep those positive affirmations coming. Offer every day for the highest good.

15. Take the time to rest deeply. Sometimes what you really need is a nap.

16. Take time out to do healthy things for yourself every day!

Chapter 9

IMPROVE IMMUNITY

Your immune cells are like a circulating nervous system. Your nervous system in fact is a circulating nervous system. It thinks. It's conscious.

—Deepak Chopra

Think of your immune system as a symphony of cells, chemicals, and organs all playing together to bring about a harmonious state of health in your body. Your immune system is also a twenty-four-hour security system, always on the alert, helping the body distinguish between itself and foreign matter and removing damaged, worn-out cells.

The Inside Scoop on Your Immune System

Your immune system doesn't have a set of organs that define it anatomically, but it does have cells throughout the body and in fact, is your body. However, the lymphatic organs—spleen, thymus, and tonsils as well as lymph nodes—play a major part.

Other systems are also integral to our immunity. The respiratory system contains lymph tissue that produces lymphocytes, the digestive system secretes acids that kill pathogens, and the urinary system contains lymph tissue that expels pathogens and maintains the body's pH balance.

Your Immune System and Germs

Germs, microorganisms that cause disease, are everywhere: in the air we breathe, the hands we shake, and in food we consume. When our immune systems are strong, it's more likely that we'll be resistant to germs that can make us sick.

Good to Know!

When the immune system is deficient, underactive, excessive, or overly reactive, it can cause autoimmune disorders. Autoimmune disorders include allergies, arthritis, asthma, Crohn's disease, diabetes, eczema, multiple sclerosis, and Parkinson's disease. Our focus should be in helping the immune system find a healthy balance.

Bacteria and Your Immune System

Bacteria are one-celled organisms, many of which are beneficial. Some, however, can cause damage by producing waste material. Illnesses caused by bacteria include diphtheria, staph, strep, tetanus, typhoid, tuberculosis, and certain forms of pneumonia. Bacteria require nutrients, oxygen, and water to survive.

Your Immune System and Viruses

Viruses are tiny particles containing RNA and DNA, too small to be seen with anything except an electron microscope. It was 1935 when viruses were discovered to be something different from bacteria. Viruses adapt easily, changing their outer coats only to resume another disguise. Viruses can't reproduce on their own and must use the reproductive capabilities of healthy cells to produce more viruses. Viral infections are usually in the body for at least a couple of days before they show up as disease.

Diseases and illnesses caused by viruses include AIDS, chicken pox, the common cold, croup, encephalitis, Epstein-Barr, flu, herpes, infectious hepatitis, kidney and bladder infections, measles, meningitis, mononucleosis, mumps, polio, rabies, some cancers, pneumonia, conjunctivitis, and tonsillitis.

How the Immune System Protects Your Body from Invaders

When your immune system is functioning at optimal levels, your body is protected from germs, bacteria, and viruses.

The Problem with Antibiotics

Each of the 100 species of common disease-causing bacteria now has at least one strain that is resistant to antibiotics. That number is rapidly increasing, becoming a major medical threat. The overuse of antibiotics (which literally means "against life") is a contributing factor in weakening the immune system. That's because antibiotics kill off helpful bacteria as well as those that are harmful.

Keep in mind that antibiotics are effective only against bacterial infections such as a sinus or urinary tract infection, not illnesses caused by viruses, such as the common cold or flu.

The Role of White Blood Cells and How They Work

White blood cells are known as leukocytes and are mainly in the vascular system but are made in the bone marrow, helping to protect the body against foreign substances. When infection occurs, white blood cell count increases as the bone marrow makes more cells, which get released into the bloodstream.

There are five types of white blood cells:

- Basophils migrate into spaces between cells and become mast cells that can produce histamine and help prevent allergic reactions. These also help control allergic reactions and inflammation.
- Eosinophils form in response to chemical contaminants and parasites. They release an enzyme that breaks down histamine.
- Lymphocytes, some of which migrate into lymphatic tissue, can become T cells in the thymus gland.
- Neutrophils seek out invaders. They contain enzymes that ingest bacteria, surround foreign matter, and discharge enzymes or devour the invader.
- Monocytes clean up cellular debris following an infection and become larger cells called macrophages.

What You Need to Know about Macrophages, Phagocytes, Lymphocytes, and T Cells

Macrophages are a type of phagocyte, a white blood cell that ingests debris and potential disease-causing organisms. Macrophages are produced in the bone marrow and digest (phagocytize) invaders (antigens), sense trouble, and send out chemical messages to attract other infection-neutralizing agents to a certain area of the body.

Macrophages travel in body parts other than the blood and are found mainly in the skin, bronchi, tonsils, appendix, breasts, and cervix. What these cells do is neutralize things that shouldn't be there, such as bacteria, parasites, viruses, chemicals, and even foreign particles.

Phagocytes

Phagocytes also include other white blood cells. A normal white blood cell count is around 4,000 to 11,000 white blood cells per cubic millimeter. Lower counts indicate weakened immunity and higher counts indicate infection.

After the macrophages partially digest some of the invader, they transfer some of that antigenic material to the B cells, which make a specific protein antibody that matches the chemical structure of the invader's protein coating.

Antibodies are Y-shaped protein molecules made by B cells. They are a mirror image of the antigen and can lock onto the antigen or invader and inactivate it. These antibodies then become known as immunoglobulins. They go to the infection site, become attached to the invader, and with the help of T cells, swallow and digest attackers. Once the body has formed a specific antibody to a specific illness, the antibody remains in the system.

Lymphocytes

Lymphocytes are white blood cells that dwell in the lymphoid tissue of the body such as the spleen, bone marrow, and tonsils as well as in lymph nodes. The other two kinds of lymphocytes are the B and T lymphocytes, both of which originate in the liver of a nine-week-old fetus and then migrate to the bone marrow.

Lymphocytes normally make up about 25 percent of the total white blood cell count. The body produces about a billion lymphocytes daily. B cells mature in the bone marrow and help produce antibody precursors that travel in search of invaders.

T Cells

T cells mature in the thymus gland and attack invaders. There are several different types of T cells, such as the following:

Killer cells attach themselves to specific cells such as bacteria, viruses, etc., and digest them.

T helpers help to stimulate killer cells and increase the body's response to the invader. They identify what needs to be eradicated in the body and stimulate cellular growth in the spleen and lymph nodes.

T-suppressor cells suppress immune response and keep the body from overreacting and attacking itself.

Interferon is found in infected cells. Healthy cells under viral attack make this protein so they can interfere with the viruses taking over.

The Thymus Gland: The Brain or Conductor of the Immune System

The thymus gland is made of two soft, pinkish lobes and lies like a bib below the thyroid gland and above the heart. It usually decreases in size after puberty and by old age can be so small that it can be difficult to identify. Other factors that decrease its size are stress, nutritional deficiency, chronic infection, and the use of steroids.

The thymus gland is responsible for the activation of T cells. It also releases polypeptide hormones, including thymosin, thymopoietin, and serum thymic factor, which all regulate many immune functions. The thymus gland is a storehouse for zinc and is rich in carotenes in its epithelial cells.

Thumping the thymus gland is a folk remedy for activating it. Perhaps that is what Tarzan was trying to do when thumping his chest before a heroic feat?

An **antibody** is a protein molecule that is produced by the immune system when it detects a harmful substance in the body called an antigen. These microorganisms include bacteria, viruses, fungi, and parasites. The antibody is carried in the blood and attracted to the specific antigen that it has been programmed to destroy.

Natural Ways to Boost Immunity

You can take many safe and natural steps to improve your immune system strength. One of the best ways is to choose the right foods, drinks, soups, and condiments to address any nutritional deficiencies that can make you prone to disease and boost immune power in many healthy ways.

Did You Know?

It's a good idea to chew your food well. That's because the salivary glands secrete enzymes that destroy bacteria, aiding your immune system.

Bone Marrow 101

Bone marrow, the soft tissue that occupies the medullary cavities of the bones, is another important part of the immune system. Immunity-producing marrow is found in the skull's flat bones and the spinal column, breastbone, collarbone, ribs, thighs, and upper arm. Stem and other immune cells are produced here.

Choose Cruciferous and High-Beta-Carotene Veggies

Include plenty of **cruciferous vegetables** such as broccoli, cabbage, and cauliflower, which are more digestible cooked and less likely to produce gas. Keep in mind that raw members of this vegetable family can inhibit thyroid function. However, high-beta-carotene vegetables such as carrots, winter squash, green leafy vegetables, and sweet potatoes strengthen the thyroid gland. These veggies also help to protect against carcinogens in the body, induce protective enzyme activity, and suppress cell-destroying free radicals.

The Value of Fermented Foods

Fermented foods such as **yogurt**, **miso** (made from soybeans), **homemade pickles**, and **unpasteurized sauerkraut** help to promote healthy intestinal flora and inhibit the growth of harmful bacteria.

Vegetables

Sea vegetables supply the body with a wide range of minerals not present in most land-grown food. Seaweeds also bind with and carry harmful chemicals and pollutants out of the body and nourish the thyroid, kidneys, bones, and teeth. Marine vegetables exhibit antibiotic, antiviral, and antifungal properties.

Shiitake mushrooms are immune enhancing, cholesterol lowering, and interferon stimulating and have been found to have antitumor activity. Another immune-enhancing mushroom to use as food or supplementation is **maitake**.

Beans such as **azuki**, **black**, and **kidney** are particularly strengthening to the kidneys, which are more prone to weakness during the cold winter season. They are also a good source of protein.

Maintain a Healthy Weight for Immune Health

Keep your weight within a healthy range for an effective immune system. Being obese has been linked to a depressed immune system.

Healthy, Immune-Boosting Foods

Rice, spelt, and **barley** are immune-strengthening grains. **Soy products** contain isoflavones, which have been shown to reduce the risk of breast and prostate cancers as well as lower cholesterol.

Chives, garlic, horseradish, leeks, scallions, and **onions** all have infection-fighting properties. To prevent garlic breath, follow your meal with a cup of peppermint tea, chew a bit of organic lemon peel, or eat the garnish of breath-freshening parsley on your plate! Chives are even a folkloric remedy to stimulate the bone marrow to produce blood.

Include infection-fighting culinary herbs in your cooking, such as **oregano, rosemary**, and **thyme**.

During winter, eat less fruit and raw salads. However, **stewed fruit** or **applesauce** with cinnamon is wonderful in colder seasons. **Steamed vegetables** would be preferable to raw ones during the cold and flu seasons. Use more **ginger** and **cayenne** to help warm you up from inside.

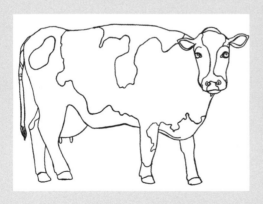

Choose Organic and Humanely Raised Protein Sources

Although it's true that we need adequate protein for effective white blood cell production, animal food such as meat and dairy contains pesticides and other harmful chemical additives that tax your immune system. Instead get your protein from organic and humanely raised animal and dairy products along with whole grains, quinoa, beans, and nuts.

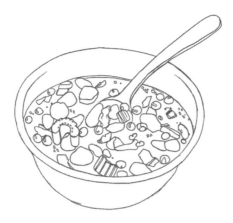

Immune-Boosting Soup

One effective and pleasant way to incorporate a number of immune-stimulating foods and herbs is to make an immune-boosting soup. You don't need to have any health problems to benefit!

- Simply sauté some chopped garlic and onions in a bit of olive oil.
- Add chopped vegetables such as broccoli, cabbage, or carrots.
- Add several sliced shiitake mushrooms.
- Add two or three pieces of astragalus slices or codonopsis and break them up into four or five pieces after they have been softened by cooking. The astragalus will be too tough and fibrous to actually eat, but it still will add therapeutic value to your broth.
- Add a small handful of sea vegetables for a host of helpful minerals.
- Add enough water to make it the consistency you desire.

Note: If you are not vegetarian, you can simmer a hormone-free chicken (with the skin removed) in your soup. It is also possible to add beans or whole grains such as barley or brown rice that have been cooked separately before adding to the soup.

After a couple of hours, take 1 teaspoon of miso for every cup (235 ml) of water that has been used in the soup. Make a paste by mixing the miso with a bit of the soup broth and then add it into the soup.

Miso is high in lecithin and helps break down fatty deposits in the body. It also helps to coat the inner wall of the colon with friendly bacteria that improves digestion, resists pathogens, and improves nutrient assimilation. Enjoy your very nutritious and delicious immune-boosting soup!

Immune-Boosting Beverages

Oat water can help strengthen the immune system and prevent infection. Simmer 2 tablespoons (10 g) of oats in a quart (946 ml) of water and simmer 30 minutes. Strain and sip as an immune tonic.

Although it's best to avoid drinking fruit juice that is excessively sweet (eat the fruit instead), occasional **cranberry juice** can be helpful in decreasing bacterial levels in the urine.

Lemon in water can provide health benefits for the immune system. When you feel an infection coming on, choose herbal teas with immune-strengthening properties.

Make a health cocktail by adding 1 tablespoon each of apple cider vinegar (15 ml) and honey (20 g) with ¼ teaspoon ginger powder stirred into a cup (235 ml) of hot water to ward off infections.

Green juices such as **wheatgrass**, **barley grass**, and **kamut grass** are high in chlorophyll, build the blood, speed up wound healing time, and help make us more resistant to infection. Also beneficial are the algaes—**chlorella**, **spirulina**, and **blue-green algae**. Chlorella has been found to be antiviral and stimulating to interferon production.

Mother Nature's News

The best food for the immune system is breast milk. If you missed out on this as an infant, you can't replace it, but at least nurse your own children so they can benefit from this perfect immune-enhancing food.

Helpful Herbs for Immune Function from A-Z

A bounty of herbs that have been tested by various world cultures over the millennia can help to boost immune health. These herbs are antimicrobial and stimulate both macrophage and T-cell activity. Your health practitioner, herbalist, naturopath, or local health food store owner can guide you in your purchase and tell you how to use each herb and what to expect.

Note: If you are pregnant or have a specific condition or health issues, talk to your health practitioner before using these herbs.

Ashwagandha: Strengthening tonic. Calms the mind. Improves exhaustion and fatigue. Adaptogen, immune stimulant, nutritive, and rejuvenative.

Astragalus: Deep immune tonic. Rich in polysaccharides. Strengthens wei chi (defense energy). Increases phagocytosis, interferon, T-cell activity, and blood cell production. Prevents atrophy of immune tissues. For autoimmune disorders. Adaptogen and chi tonic.

Baptisia: High in polysaccharides that increase phagocytosis. For both lymphatic swelling and deep inflammation. Antiseptic and surface immune tonic.

Black walnut leaves, nut, bark: Contains juglone, which has activity against candida, staph, and strep. Alterative, antifungal, anti-inflammatory, and antiseptic.

Boneset: Increases resistance to bacterial and viral infections. Used to break up fevers, colds, and flu. Immune enhancing by inducing sweating so that toxins are eliminated through the skin. Diaphoretic, febrifuge, immune stimulant, and tonic.

Burdock root, seed: Antiseptic and antifungal due to polyacetylenes. Bone marrow tonic. Adaptogen, alterative, anti-inflammatory, diaphoretic, nutritive, and rejuvenative.

Cat's claw: Activates macrophages, lymphocytes, and leukocytes. Inhibits blood platelet aggregation. Antifungal, anti-inflammatory, antioxidant, antiseptic, and antiviral.

Cayenne: High in vitamin C. Stimulates endorphin production. Alterative, anti-inflammatory, antibiotic, antioxidant, antiseptic, antiviral, carminative, and circulatory tonic.

Codonopsis: Deep immune tonic. Helps build red blood cells. Enhances transformation of white blood cells into T cells. For autoimmune disorders. Strengthens weak systems. Tonifies kidneys and adrenals. Adaptogen, chi tonic, and nutritive.

Dandelion root: Improves spleen function. Antifungal, anti-inflammatory, and antiseptic.

Echinacea: High in polysaccharides. Stimulates interferon production and helper T cells. Inhibits hyaluronidase, making cells more resistant to pathogens. Increases activity of phagocytes and macrophages. For acute infections. Alterative antifungal, antiseptic.

Eleuthero: Increases T-helper cells and enhances white blood cells. Improves nonspecific resistance to disease. Reduces cell inflammation and improves endurance. Adaptogen, anti-inflammatory, and chi tonic.

Garlic: Kills a wide range of disease-causing organisms including viruses, bacteria, fungi, and protozoans. Increases body's resistance to infection. Protects against epidemics. Surface immune herb. Alterative, antioxidant, immune stimulant, and vasodilator.

Ginseng Asian, American: Bone marrow tonic that restores production of cells. Enhances phagocytosis and increases immunoglobulins. Promotes lymphocytic transformation and production of red and white blood cells. Contains germanium. Adaptogen, chi tonic, and digestive tonic.

Goldenseal: Surface immune herb. Reduces infection in mucous membranes. Stimulates circulation to the spleen and activates macrophages. Contains berberine, which stimulates macrophage activity. Active against a wide range of pathogens. Alterative, antifungal, anti-inflammatory, antiseptic, antiviral, and bitter tonic.

Lemon balm: Antiviral, carminative, diaphoretic, digestive tonic, nervine, and rejuvenative.

Lemongrass: Shows activity against gram-positive bacteria. Antiseptic, antiviral, diaphoretic, and digestive tonic.

Licorice: Inhibits viral growth and inactivates virus particles. Increases number of antibodies and efficiency of white blood cells. Stimulates production of interferon, slows tumor growth, and improves adrenal health. Anti-inflammatory, antiseptic, and chi tonic.

Myrrh: Surface immune herb. Increases both the number and motility of white blood cells. Normalizes mucous membrane activity and inhibits infection. Alterative, anti-inflammatory, antifungal, antiseptic, carminative, decongestant, and rejuvenative.

Nettle: Rich in chlorophyll. Natural antihistamine. Strengthens kidneys and spleen. Alterative, circulatory stimulant, nutritive, and tonic.

P'au d'arco: Contains lapachol, which has been found effective against gram-positive, acid-fast bacteria and fungi. Increases red blood cells. Deep immune herb. Antifungal, alterative, anti-inflammatory, antioxidant, antiseptic, antiviral, and immune stimulant.

Propolis: Effective against bacteria, virus, and fungi. Strengthens the thyroid and thymus glands. Rich in flavonoids. Enhances white blood cell activity.

Reishi: Deep immune tonic. Improves cellular immunity. Immunoregulator. Stimulates phagocytosis and increases resistance to bacterial, parasitic, and viral infection. Inhibits histamine and activates interferon. Adaptogen, anti-inflammatory, and antiseptic.

Schizandra: Decreases fatigue and increase the body's resistance to infection. Improves oxygen metabolism. For bone marrow regeneration, liver protection.

Shiitake: Bone marrow tonic. Rich in polysaccharides. Stimulates activity of macrophages, interferon, and natural killer cells. Adaptogen, antiviral, immune stimulant, kidney and liver tonic, rejuvenative, and restorative.

Thyme: Helps deter bacterial, fungal, and viral infections. Antifungal, antiseptic, diaphoretic, rejuvenative, tonic, and vulnerary.

Usnea: Usnic acid has been found more effective than penicillin against staph and strep. Usnic acid disrupts their ability to produce energy, and they die. Herbal broad-spectrum antibiotic. Surface immune herb. Antifungal, antiseptic, and immune stimulant.

Beta-Carotene and Vitamin A

Both beta-carotene and vitamin A can help strengthen our immune systems by improving the health of our mucous membranes, making us more resistant to airborne and intestinal invaders. These nutrients are also believed to stimulate the thymus gland to produce T cells needed in preventing infection.

Vitamin A helps killer cells digest invaders. Diets high in beta-carotene appear to help make us more resistant to cancers of the cervix, colon, lung, prostate, and stomach. Both nutrients help to make an enzyme called lysozyme that attacks germs landing on mucous membranes.

B Vitamins

Taking a B-complex vitamin can help your body stay well. Vitamin B_1 works as an antioxidant and preserves the potency of T cells. A B_1 deficiency can lead to a decrease in B- and T-cell production.

B_2 and B_6 aid in the production of antibodies that fight infection. B_6 helps increase white blood cell production.

B_{12} and folic acid are needed for the production of white blood cells and lymphocyte activity. Folic acid enhances T cells' ability to digest invaders.

Panothenic acid reduces histamine response. It also nourishes and protects the adrenal glands and promotes antibody production.

Niacin (B_3) dilates blood vessels, which may help leukocytes to move through blood vessel walls.

Vitamin C

The sunshine vitamin is also an antioxidant that strengthens the body's resistance to infection. Vitamin C helps protect white blood cells, boosts macrophage activity, and raises interferon levels as well as thymic hormones and antibody levels. Vitamin C also helps to detoxify histamine.

Because our skin is one of our first lines of defense, vitamin C is needed for collagen production and wound healing (see sidebar on page 143 for more advice on taking care of your skin).

Bioflavonoids

Taking vitamin C with bioflavonoids can also help the body resist infection. Bioflavonoids have antiviral activity and improve the effectiveness of vitamin C. Quercetin, also part of the C complex, has antiviral activity. Pycnogenol has anti-inflammatory properties and helps to transport vitamin C.

Vitamin E is an antioxidant and free-radical scavenger that increases helper T cells and antibody response. It also strengthens the membranes of macrophages.

Immune-Boosting Minerals

Many minerals can help improve immune function. For example, **selenium**, an antioxidant, is necessary for antibody production and potentiates phagocytes to kill bacteria. **Germanium** has antiviral and antitumor activity. It's also an antioxidant that helps activate macrophages and killer cells.

Magnesium produces properdin, a blood protein that helps fight viruses and bacteria. It also helps prevent thymus gland atrophy and improves phagocytosis.

Zinc has been found to have inhibiting effects on viral replication. It also helps increase natural killer cell activity in smokers. Zinc nourishes the thymus gland, which will shrink if zinc is deficient. Zinc also produces histamine, which dilates capillaries so that white blood cells can rush to the area of infection.

More Nutrients for Better Immune Health

Not getting enough **coenzyme Q$_{10}$** is linked to an impaired immune function. You need it to boost the activity of immune cells.

Glutathione is an antioxidant that helps to neutralize and get rid of free radicals. If its levels are low, T cells cannot function.

Taking **probiotics** such as **acidophilus** as a supplement can help inhibit candida, which contributes to a weakened immune system.

L-arginine increases lymphocyte activity in the blood. It can help improve immune functions that have been compromised by disease and/or surgery.

Are You Missing These Two Nutrients?

Not getting enough copper and iron can diminish immune function. You need copper for antibody production, and an iron deficiency can make you more prone to infection and decrease the number of B and T lymphocytes.

L-cysteine is a sulfur-containing amino acid that helps in the production of antibodies. The liver uses it to detoxify chemicals and pollutants that can weaken the immune system.

L-lysine has antiviral properties.

L-phenylalanine, if deficient, can make antibodies less effective.

Use Aromatherapy to Boost Immunity

Essential oils can help improve immunity when used in the bath, in diffusers, or in massage. Consider the antiviral properties of **cinnamon**, **garlic**, **oregano**, **tea tree**, and **thyme**. Both **patchouli** and **tea tree oil** have antifungal properties.

Antibacterial essential oils include **balsam of Peru**, **bergamot**, **cinnamon**, **cedarwood**, **clove**, **lavender**, **lemon**, **orange**, **oregano**, **pine**, **tea tree**, and **thyme**. Antiseptic properties are found in essential oils of **clary sage**, **grapefruit**, **lemon**, **lime**, **marjoram**, and **sage**.

The Effect of Stress on Your Immune System

When we are stressed, fatigued, and under-nourished, our immune system has a difficult time doing its job. Stress is one of the greatest hazards for the immune system, as it inhibits interferon production. Emotions associated with a weakened immune system include anxiety, bereavement (see chapter 11), depression, guilt, isolation, loss, and loneliness.

Meditation, prayer, and inspirational readings are all good ways to relieve stress. Practice right living, positive thinking, and healthy relation-ships for a healthy immune system. Be aware of negative thoughts and answer them with a more constructive view. Have creative outlets and a job you enjoy. Avoid disciplines so rigid that they stress you out. For more ways to relieve stress, see chapter 2.

Take Care of the Skin You're In

The skin is often referred to as one of our first lines of defense, because it serves as a barrier to possible invaders and its natural oil content helps to inacti-vate microbes. Take care of small wounds; use a daily supplement of **fish or hemp seed oil**, which has immune-enhancing, T-cell-activating, and anti-inflam-matory properties so the skin will be well lubricated; practice dry brush skin massaging; wear natural-fiber clothing that is not constricting; and sleep in natural-fiber bedding so the skin can breathe.

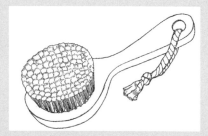

Important Advice for Improving Immunity

1. **Use cold water in the shower.** If you feel brave, try ending your showers with cold water. This constricts blood vessels on the surface, sending blood deeper into the body, facilitating the removal of toxins, and increasing the production of T-cells.

2. **During inclement weather dress warm.** It is especially important to protect the kidneys, head, and feet. Overexposure to wind and temperature extremes can also weaken the immune system.

3. **Sunbathing can suppress the immune system** for up to fifteen days and decrease lymphocyte activity.

4. **Consider removing mercury fillings** and doing it right. Exposure to heavy metals can weaken the immune system by inhibiting antibody response and T-cell activity. Minimize your chemical exposure.

5. **Removing organs unnecessarily,** such as the tonsils and appendix, which are part of the immune system, can increase stress on the rest of the immune system.

6. **Take care of minor infections** so that big ones don't have to clamor for your attention.

7. **Get enough sleep.** During sleep immune-specific chemicals are released in the body. You'll find more information in chapter 5.

Skip This!

Exposure to radiation destroys B cells. Overexposure to electromagnetic pollution may also have an adverse effect upon the immune system. Avoid having your sleeping area contaminated by electric blankets, water bed heaters, digital clocks, and other electronic paraphernalia.

8. **Find ways to stay active.** Get outside and enjoy sports or just tromp around. Yoga, chi kung, and tai chi can be done indoors during any kind of weather. Exercise, but not to exhaustion. Practice deep breathing! Dance!

9. **Practice visualization.** See yourself in good health and well-being.

10. **Allow yourself to rest and recover.** We can't always avoid every cold that comes our way. When you can, give yourself the opportunity to rest, recover, and nurture yourself to wellness.

Chapter 10

REDUCE CHRONIC PAIN

One word frees us of all the weight and pain in life.
That word is love.
— Sophocles

One hundred million people in the United States suffer pain daily. Pain is Nature's way of giving us clues to our body's ailments so that we can do something about them. But that doesn't mean that it's easy to deal with. Chronic pain, especially, can be difficult both mentally and emotionally. Natural remedies can provide relief from mild to moderate pain and make way for healing. If your pain does not abate, however, it's important to see your health care practitioner.

What Causes Pain?

Pain is often due to inflammation, which is a protective function that prevents bacteria, toxins, and foreign material at the site of an injury from spreading. When tissues are injured, they release chemicals like histamine that irritate the nerves. Histamine begins the inflammatory process, dilating blood vessels, which increases their permeability so the healing can begin. Kinins are proteins in blood that dilate blood vessels, also increasing their permeability, and attract white blood cells to the inflamed site.

The Power of Prostaglandins

Prostaglandins result when arachadonic acid (a fatty acid) breaks down, then COX-1 and COX-2 enzymes form, contributing to more inflammation by intensifying the kinin and histamine effects.

COX-1 is present in our tissues on a regular basis and produces prostaglandins that help regulate normal body functions. COX-2 is not normally present and is produced only at the sites of inflammation, where it helps in prostaglandin production that increases inflammation.

Other chemicals that contribute to pain when you are injured are eicosanoids (prostaglandins, leukotrienes, thromboxanes, and platelet activating factor). Substance P is a peptide that exists mainly in the spinal cord, binds to pain receptors in the brain and spinal cord, and directly produces pain.

Pain messages travel up from the spinal cord to the thalamus (base of the brain), where they meet a second synapse. One way that our brain responds to pain is by producing morphine-like hormones known as endorphins. After this crossing, the pain message then travels to the brain's cerebral cortex.

Necessary Nutrients

Of course, the best way to relieve pain is to eliminate the underlying problem. Although this isn't always possible, choosing certain foods can have a soothing effect by affecting our perception of pain.

Whole grains (millet, black rice, buckwheat, amaranth, and quinoa), poultry, and raw dairy products, for example, are high in the naturally occurring amino acid tryptophan, which encourages production of the calming neurotransmitter serotonin.

Good to Know!

In holistic medicine all pain is considered stagnant energy. Superficial pain originates in the nerves of the skin. Pain that originates from deeper structures such as the muscles, joints, and tendons is considered deep pain. Pain from the organs is called visceral pain.

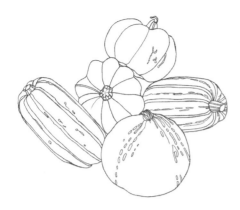

Foods That Ease Pain

Some particularly beneficial foods for someone suffering from pain include oats, corn, brown rice, black-eyed peas, broccoli, cauliflower, cherries, pineapple, grapes, winter squashes, sesame seeds, turmeric, rosemary, ginger, sage, green tea, olive oil, and flaxseeds.

Bromelain, an enzyme that comes from the stem and juice of pineapples, reduces inflammatory prostaglandins. Research shows that bromelain and quercetin work better together. Take 2,000 mg of bromelain divided into two doses and 500 mg of quercetin two times a day. Contraindications are pregnancy, bleeding disorder, and uncontrolled blood pressure.

Cayenne pepper, such as that found in chili, helps to stimulate endorphin production. Strawberries, which contain natural salicylates, are cooling and anti-inflammatory. Raw string beans have long been considered a therapeutic food for arthritis for their ability to eliminate uric acid, which can contribute to joint pain. Celery seed as a condiment helps eliminate uric acid in the body, too.

Eat Tart Cherries!

Research at the Oregon Health and Science University showed that tart cherry juice has the highest anti-inflammatory content of any food and can help people with osteoarthritis manage their condition better. Cherries contain antioxidants called anthocyanins, which give them their red color and help reduce inflammation. In a study of twenty women ages forty to seventy who had osteoarthritis, the researchers found that drinking tart cherry juice twice daily for three weeks helped reduce inflammation markers. You can eat tart cherries fresh, dried, or frozen to receive benefits or take a supplement: 500 mg four times a day or drink tart cherry juice twice daily for three weeks. For more information visit www.choosecherries.com.

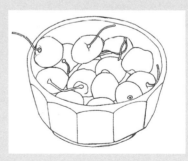

Eat Fish!

Seafood, especially cod, halibut, tuna, flounder, striped bass, salmon, and herring, helps relieve pain because it contains a neurotoxin that helps to block the neurological transmission or pain signals to the muscles. Research in the medical journal *Surgical Neurology* in 2006 showed that omega-3 fatty acids found in fish oil reduce the inflammatory response, and as a result, pain, with no significant side effects. The dose that proved most effective is 2 to 4 grams of DHA and EPA. Take 1,500 to 3,000 mg total fat per day—the lower end for maintenance and the higher end for more acute flare-ups of pain and stiffness.

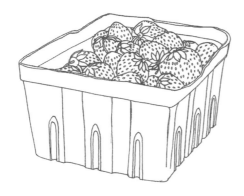

Topical Treatments

Treatments that can be used topically include castor oil, charcoal poultices, hot ginger tea (see sidebar on ginger on page 150), salt packs (heat salt in a pan and put into cotton pillowcase), and cold mashed tofu.

Topricin, a homeopathic cream, provides soothing relief for many different types of mild to moderate pain. Mustard foot baths are an old-time remedy to draw the blood away from an injured area.

Supplements That Can Help Ease Pain

If you have chronic pain, chances are you reach for NSAIDs, nonsteroidal anti-inflammatory drugs like aspirin, ibuprofen, and celecoxib (Celebrex), to block the enzymes that trigger inflammation and pain. Unfortunately, that relief can come at a high cost with side effects such as ulcers, high blood pressure, and even heart attacks and strokes, according to a recent study in the medical journal *The Lancet*.

Natural cures work in a way similar to NSAIDs but are a safer alternative when it comes to easing the pain and inflammation of chronic conditions, from arthritis to fibromyalgia. Home remedies can also cost less than prescription or over-the-counter medicines and can have fewer side effects.

But before you try these remedies discuss possible side effects and contraindications with your doctor. Make an appointment with an integrative physician or osteopathic doctor who is open to alternative cures.

Healing Herbs

Many of the herbs that help pain are classified as anesthetics, which numb existing pain either locally or generally. Analgesics help to allay pain when used internally without disturbing consciousness. Anodynes are sedating and help keep pain from being perceived by the brain.

Cayenne: Stimulates endorphin production. For arthritis, headache, migraine, pain, and shingles. Topically, it blocks transmission of substance P, which transports pain messages to the brain. A study published in the *Journal of Rheumatology* in 1992 showed that capsaicin (the key ingredient in cayenne pepper) relieves the tenderness and pain of osteoarthritis.

Make your own topical treatment by steeping 1 tablespoon (5.3 g) of cayenne in 1 pint (475 ml) of apple cider vinegar. You can also buy capsaicin cream at your health food store.

Chamomile: A good herb for people with various complaints. For migraine, neuralgia, pain, stress, and ulcers. Nervine and sedative.

Cloves: Good for stomachache. Applied topically to numb pain, such as toothaches. Analgesic and anesthetic.

Corydalis: Helps relieve pain from traumatic injury. The alkaloid tetrahydropalmatine appears to block dopamine receptors in the nervous system. Used for backache, dysmenorrhea, headache, and rheumatism.

Skip This!

Do your best to avoid vasodilating substances, which can cause swelling in the blood vessels and therefore pain. Foods that are potentiators of pain include yeasts, processed meats (hot dogs, bologna, etc.), aged cheese, the additive MSG, and alcohol. Some of the above foods also contain the amino acid tyramine, which causes vasoconstriction.

Sip This!

Green tea contains polyphenols, a type of antioxidant that cools the inflammation of rheumatoid arthritis. Research at the University of Michigan Health System in 2007 showed that this compound may inhibit the production of molecules that cause the destruction of cartilage and bone. Drink four cups of green tea a day or take an EGCG (active ingredient in green tea) supplement: 2,000 mg two times a day.

Spice Spotlight: Ginger

This popular spice contains powerful phenolic compounds and antioxidants such as shogoals, zingerone, and gingerols, which can help to reduce pain and inflammation. A review published in the *Journal of Medicinal Food* showed that ginger, like NSAIDs, inhibits the COX-1 and -2 enzymes that cause inflammation.

A study conducted at the Miami Veterans Affairs Medical Center and the University of Miami in 2001 showed that a highly purified and standardized ginger extract was effective in reducing the symptoms of knee osteoarthritis.

Ginger compresses can be very comforting for painful conditions. Just dip a clean washcloth into a cup of hot (not scalding) ginger tea and apply to the aching joint in question. Cover with a dry cloth to help hold the heat in until it's cool. Replace as needed. You can also use topical creams that contain ginger to ease pain and inflammation and reduce stiffness.

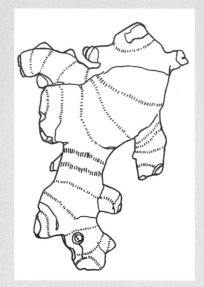

Cramp bark: Analgesic, anti-inflammatory, antispasmodic, nervine, sedative. Used for postpartum pain, rheumatism, and spasms of legs and lower back. Found in liniments for arthritic joints, sore muscles, and back pain.

Feverfew: Inhibits certain prostaglandins and prevents blood platelet aggregation. Used on a regular basis to prevent migraines. Helpful for arthritis, headache, pain, and rheumatism.

Frankincense: This inhibits the COX enzyme pathway and reduces inflammatory prostaglandins. Used topically to relieve joint pain. Liniment and salve for sports injuries and arthritis pain. Analgesic, antispasmodic, nervine.

Hops: Sedative to parasympathetic nervous system. Helps headache, insomnia, pain, restlessness, stomachache, and stress. Muscle relaxant, nervine, sedative, and soporific.

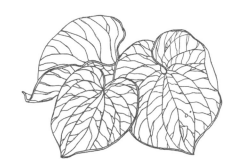

Kava kava: Both a skeletal and muscle relaxant as well as a central nervous system depressant. Helps anxiety, cramps, depression, dysmenorrhea, insomnia, neuralgia, pain, and rheumatism. Analgesic, antispasmodic, sedative, and tonic.

Passionflower: Slows breakdown of serotonin and norepinephrine. Depresses the motor side of the spinal column. For headache, insomnia, muscle spasms, neuralgia, shingles, and stress. Anti-inflammatory, antispasmodic, nervine, and sedative.

Skullcap: Sedates the brain and spinal column. Encourages endorphin production. Helpful for arthritis, headache, neuralgia, rheumatism, and spasms. Nervine and sedative.

Stinging nettle: The stinging part of the nettle draws blood to the joint, relieving pain and inflammation. If you're feeling brave, striking the inflamed joint with a fresh cutting from a nettle plant helps relieve joint pain. But an easier way is to take this as a supplement. Capsules can cause stomach upset, so drink it as a tea or use it topically on the area that is painful.
Note: Pregnant woman should not take it.

Saint-John's-wort: For nerve and spinal pain. Helps heal damaged nerves when used internally and topically. Used for dysmenorrhea, neuralgia, and rheumatism. Anti-inflammatory, antispasmodic, nervine, sedative, and vulnerary.

Turmeric: Contains two natural compounds, curcumin and curcuminoids, that decrease inflammation naturally. A study in the medical journal *Arthritis and Rheumatism* in 2006 showed that turmeric may be effective in helping to relieve symptoms of rheumatoid arthritis.

Valerian: This is a smooth muscle and skeletal relaxant as well as a central nervous system depressant. For headache, migraine, neuralgia, shingles, stress, and trauma. Nervine and sedative. Warming.

Vervain: Helps dysmenorrhea, migraine, neuralgia, stress, and general pain. Contains verbenalin, a tranquilizing glucoside. Anti-inflammatory, antispasmodic, nervine, sedative, vasoconstrictor, and vulnerary.

White willow: Contains salicin. Inhibits prostaglandin production. For arthritis, backache, headache, joint inflammation, migraine, rheumatism, and general pain. Analgesic, anti-inflammatory, antirheumatic, and tonic. Cooling.

Wild lettuce: General pain and restlessness. Believed to inhibit the spinal column's referral of pain. Analgesic, sedative.

Wild yam: Moves congested chi. Use for arthritis, muscle cramps and spasms, neuralgia, ovarian pain, and rheumatism. Anti-inflammatory, antirheumatic, antispasmodic, and sedative.

Wood betony: Helps headache, migraine, neuralgia, pain, and stress. Analgesic, antispasmodic, cerebral tonic, circulatory stimulant, nervine, sedative, and vulnerary.

Well-Being Supplements

If you're suffering from pain, certain supplements can help. Both **vitamin B₁** and **calcium** are thought to raise one's pain threshold. **Vitamins C** and **E** are necessary for the production of endorphins. Magnesium can relax muscle spasms while omega-3 fatty acids reduce inflammation and inhibit unfriendly prostaglandin production.

Vitamin D is also helpful in managing pain. A study published in the medical journal *Pain Medicine* in 2009 showed a link between low levels of vitamin D and the amount of narcotic medications needed by chronic pain patients. Mayo Clinic researchers found that those who had low levels of vitamin D needed nearly twice as much medication as those who had enough.

Your health practitioner can check your vitamin D levels. This is especially important if you have fibromyalgia and bone and joint pain. If you are deficient, she may recommend that you take a supplement for natural pain relief.

If you have osteoarthritis, you may find natural pain relief by supplementing with **SAM-e**.

Research shows that it may be as effective as painkillers like Celebrex. However, using SAM-e isn't cheap. Expect to pay between $80 and $120 out of pocket. **MSM (methylsulfonylmethane)** may also help relieve osteopathic pain.

DLPA is made from one of the essential amino acids, phenylalanine. Phenylalanine inhibits enkephalinase, an enzyme that breaks down enkephalins and endorphins, so that the naturally occurring endorphins can survive longer. DLPA helps relieve chronic pain yet does not block the nerve transmission of short-term acute pain. In other words, if you touch a hot stove, you will still know it immediately and quickly move yourself away.

Most people obtain relief within one to four weeks when using DLPA. Although DLPA is considered very safe, it should not be used with MAO-inhibiting drugs (some types of antidepressants), during pregnancy, or by phenylketonurics. Another benefit of DLPA is that some people who suffer from chronic pain are able to use it for a couple of weeks and then go off it for the next two weeks, yet have pain-relieving benefits that last all month long.

Good to Know!

Tea tree oil from the leaves of the *Melaleuca alternifolia* tree is helpful when it comes to reducing inflammation. Buy it in your health food store and use it topically to reduce inflammation.

Enzyme supplementation (check out Wobenzyme) reduces inflammation and is very effective. One capsule is taken three times daily between meals. Glucosamine is a compound that naturally occurs in the body, a glucose molecule bonded to the amino acid glutamine. It helps repair and/or preserve cartilage tissue and also enhance hyaluronic acid, the compound that lubricates and absorbs shock-absorbing properties of the fluid that bathes the joints. (Take 1,500 mg daily.)

Glucosamine sulphate and chondroitin taken together reduce inflammation and help to repair traumatized tissue and lubricate and cushion joints. They're effective for moderate knee osteoarthritis. Take a supplement of 1,500 mg glucosamine and 1,200 mg chondroitin. MSM helps to promote tissue repair in the body by providing sulfur.

If You Have Diabetic Neuropathy

Research published in the medical journal *Drugs in R&D* in 2002 showed that acetyl-L-carnitine is helpful in easing diabetic nerve pain. Alpha-lipoic acid can help with diabetic neuropathy as well, reducing pain and slowing nerve damage, along with improving insulin sensitivity.

Thrifty Cures

Throbbing pain, or when it hurts too much to touch, like a banged nose or finger, is best relieved by a cold application, such as an ice pack or cool compress. Sharp pain, on the other hand, is often best remedied by heat such as a hot water bottle or hot compress. Or brew up a pot of herbal tea and use it to make herbal compresses and apply topically.

Natural Practices and Holistic Therapies to Ease Pain

The Power of Yoga

Exercise helps to stimulate feel-good endorphin production, which can ease the perception and feeling of pain. In fact, according to a review of research between 2010 and 2013 published in the *Journal of Evidence-Based Complementary and Alternative Medicine*, practitioners of yoga had less pain (see the sidebar on yoga for migraines on page 158) and morning stiffness, were able to be more active, and were less stressed and depressed, with a better perspective on life.

Acupuncture also helps stimulate endorphin production. Research in the medical journal *Complementary Therapies in Medicine* (2007) indicates that acupuncture provides 50 to 80 percent relief to people with acute or chronic pain. In Traditional Chinese Medicine, it is thought to relieve the stagnation of chi, or energy, in the body. To find a practitioner visit the American Association of Acupuncture and Oriental Medicine at www.aaaomonline.org.

Aromatherapy

Essential oils like wintergreen salicin, a pain-relieving compound. Citrus oils like lemon and orange are calming and anti-inflammatory.

Other best bets include birch, cajuput, camphor, chamomile, coriander, eucalyptus, fir, frankincense, geranium, ginger, lavender, peppermint, pine, and rosemary. Put it a diffuser to fill the room with soothing scents or use these oils in diluted form for massaging the painful area.

 Cure Caution:

DMSO is a controversial substance, but some have found it helpful for pain. DMSO (dimethyl sulfoxide) is actually a solvent by-product from the paper-making industry. It has been prescribed for pain in Russia since 1971. DMSO passes through the tissue, relieves pain, reduces swelling, is a muscle relaxant, has bacteriostatic properties, increases circulation, is analgesic, and can help soften scar tissue. Negative side effects include garlic breath, irritated skin, and blurry vision. Best bet? Try other, safer natural remedies.

Take a Bath

Epsom salt is high in magnesium, which soothes and relaxes stiff joints and muscles. Soaking in a warm bath to which a pound (455 g) of Epsom salts and five to ten drops of a pain-relieving essential oil has been added releases toxins and relieves pain.

You can also take a magnesium glycinate supplement (best absorption, fewer side effects) for chronic pain. Take 400 to 600 mg a day. Increase as needed to bowel tolerance.

Relax and Ease Pain with Progressive Relaxation

Progressive relaxation eases pain by triggering the relaxation response. Pioneered by Herbert Benson, M.D., at the Benson-Henry Institute for Mind Body Medicine at Massachusetts General Hospital in Boston, it enhances the body's own morphinelike substances in what is referred to as the runner's high.

It's easy to do. Just lie down (if you can), think of each body part, flex, and then relax it. Start with your face and move downward through your whole body, from your shoulders to your toes. Do it once or twice a day for 10 to 20 minutes on a regular basis for best results. For more information, visit www.bensonhenryinstitute.org.

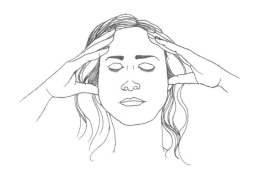

Natural Remedies for the Pain of Migraine Headaches

If you're one of the 30 million people in the United States who suffer from migraine headaches, then you know all about the intense, debilitating, pulsating, throbbing pain that they cause. Migraines can also result in light and noise sensitivity, nausea, and vomiting. The pain is usually located on one side but it may shift from side to side.

Research shows that natural remedies can help reduce the frequency and the intensity of migraines. Start with one remedy and gradually add the others to see if they can help you. You'll need to be patient, though; it takes on average two to three months for these to work.

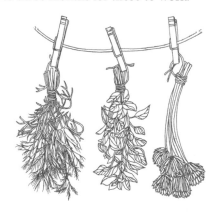

Butterbur, a member of the daisy family, reduces inflammation in brain blood vessels, relieving pressure on surrounding nerves. It was used by Native Americans as a remedy for headache and inflammation. Today it is widely used to prevent and reduce the intensity of migraines. A study in the medical journal *Neurology* (2004) showed butterbur can reduce the frequency of migraines by almost half. It also reduces the intensity and length of migraines.

To prevent migraines, take 50 mg butterbur root extract daily. Get a brand that is free of a toxic substance called pyrrolizidine alkaloids. One of the best brands of butterbur rhizome extract is Petadolex, made by Weber & Weber. If you sense a migraine is about to occur, take 150 mg of **Migravent**, a product that helps prevent migraines, contains butterbur.

Supplementing with **magnesium** relaxes blood vessels and reduces the likelihood that migraine-inducing electric signals in the brain will be generated. You can take magnesium by itself to prevent migraines (200 mg each evening) or take a combination formula. **Migre-Lief** prevents migraines with a combination of magnesium, vitamin B$_2$, and feverfew. Take it once day for at least a month before you expect to see results.

Vitamin B$_2$ may be as effective as beta-blockers, a therapy traditionally used to prevent migraines, because it relaxes blood vessels, according to research in the journal *Neurology*. Other studies show that B$_2$ can decrease migraine frequency by 67 percent after just six weeks. You'll need to take daily doses of 400 mg of B$_2$ each morning for at least a month to expect to see a reduction in migraine frequency.

Good to Know!

1. Three-quarters of migraine sufferers are women.

2. Most migraine sufferers are between ages twenty and forty-five.

3. Migraines run in families, so if your parents have migraines, chances are, you may have them, too.

4. Migraines may occur cyclically or from a particular food allergy.

5. Yeasted breads, gluten-rich foods, citrus fruits, and processed meats can also bring on migraines.

6. Menstrual cycles and birth control pills may be a factor.

Research shows that migraine headaches may result from disruption of energy production in the body. **CoQ$_{10}$** is a nutrient that plays an important role in the energy that each cell needs to function.

Research published in *Cephalalgia: An International Journal of Headache* (2002) showed that when thirty-two patients (twenty-six women, six men) with a history of migraines were treated with CoQ$_{10}$, 61 percent of patients had a greater than 50 percent reduction in the number of days with migraine headache. Best of all, there were no side effects.

Enzymatic Therapy makes a good CoQ$_{10}$ supplement. Alternatively, get the best that you can afford. Take 400 mg each day.

Feverfew, like butterbur, is a member of the daisy family and helps to stop blood platelets from releasing too much serotonin and histamine, both of which can dilate blood vessels and lead to migraines. A systematic review of research in the medical journal *Public Health Nutrition* (2000) showed that feverfew is effective and safe in the prevention of migraines.

The dried leaves, flowers, and stems of feverfew are used to make supplements found in capsules, tablets, and extracts. It's important to buy high-quality supplements especially when it comes to nutrients like feverfew, to ensure botanical integrity. A good high-potency brand is MygraFew by Nature's Way. Feverfew works best as a preventive taken on a daily basis rather than when a headache is already in progress.

Research shows that homeopathic feverfew can also help reduce the frequency of migraines. Ask your holistic doctor what is right for you.

Note: Pregnant women should not use feverfew.

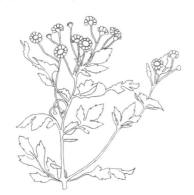

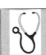

When to See Your M.D.

If your headaches have gotten worse over days and weeks, if you've never had headaches before (especially if you are over fifty), or if the headaches come on suddenly and don't go away, call your doctor. Other warning signs include weakness, numbness, or a change in your hearing, sight, memory, personality, or cognitive abilities. Also contact your doctor if your headache is accompanied by a stiff neck, rash, nausea, vomiting, fever, breathing problems, or a head injury.

Brigitte's Advice for Soothing Pain and Discomfort

1. I've found that many people can tolerate pain better if they have friends watching them, or if there is some kind of reward.

2. Practice deep, slow breathing. Visualize yourself inhaling healing light and exhaling the pain out of your body.

3. The color **blue** is considered anti-inflammatory. Some people have found that exposure to blue light, visualizing breathing in the color blue, or simply wearing blue helps them to feel calm.

4. Tightening the area around where the pain is centered and then releasing can help to alleviate pain as an exercise.

5. Some people find it helpful to write about their experience with pain in a journal. This may even help you to find clues, such as pain is lessened on the days when you take a walk.

6. You can use art to describe your pain by drawing it. Is it like a biting dog or burning flames? In your mind's eye, gently muzzle the dog or pour water on the fire. Next, draw images that soothe pain and visualize them to find relief.

7. Most importantly, be kind and gentle with yourself. See chapter 2 for ways to be good to you.

Yoga for Migraines

A study in *Headache* (2007) showed the effectiveness of yoga therapy in managing migraines. Seventy-two patients with migraines without aura were randomly assigned to yoga therapy or a self-care group for three months. At the end of the study, headache frequency, severity, pain, and associated depression and anxiety were all significantly lower in the yoga therapy group compared to the self-care group.

Choose a type of yoga that you feel comfortable with. Good practices for beginners include Kripalu yoga, viniyoga, or gentle yoga. Find a teacher who will gently guide you through the poses.

You'll also find CDs so you can do slow yoga at home. *Yoga Journal* online features videos to show you how to do different poses correctly and how to build a sequence. You can also download (for a fee) instructional yoga videos to help you reduce stress and sleep better, and even desk yoga so you can stay relaxed and balanced at work! Visit www.yogajournal.com.

Yoga nidra or yogic sleep can also help reduce stress that can trigger migraines. For more information visit chapter 2 in this book.

Chapter 11

RECOVER FROM GRIEF AND TRAUMA

What soap is for the body, tears are for the soul.
—Anonymous

An essential part of learning to live more harmoniously and happily is learning how to deal with and accept loss: how to let go, recover, and ultimately move on. The same goes if you experience any type of trauma. The process from any event to healing and life afterward can be a bumpy road. So is recovery from any addiction. These natural remedies can help.

Growing through Grief

Every human being experiences grief. Grief helps us appreciate what is important and realize what we may have taken for granted. Common reasons for deep grief can be death and the ending of a relationship. If you are the one being left, loss and separation can cause feelings similar to death of a loved one.

Sometimes ending a short-term relationship can be more painful than a long one, because in a short relationship, you still hold hopes and expectations. In a long-term relationship, you most likely have had time to see what hasn't been working. People change. Accept this as a challenge to find new opportunities.

The Effect of Grief on the Body

When you are grieving, your heart rate, blood pressure, and hydrochloric acid production rise. It is not unusual to experience a sensation of numbness, pain along the breastbone, and sinus congestion when grieving.

Sorrow can cause increased adrenaline production, which runs along a path from the lower cerebellum, through the pituitary gland, to the adrenals. Sorrow can accelerate hardening of the cerebral arteries, causing coronary arteriosclerosis. Grief can cause broken spasmodic breathing, where you sob easily.

If grief is severe and continues, it can be a contributing factor in heart disease and arteriosclerosis. Being grief stricken for extended periods can lead to a weakened immunity.

Traditional Chinese Medicine: Grief

In Traditional Chinese Medicine (TCM), the Metal Element, associated with the lungs and large intestines, is connected to the emotion of grief. Sadness can cause a depletion of chi, contribute to chronic fatigue, and increase susceptibility to lung problems.

According to TCM, there are four forms of sorrow:

1. Grievous sorrow, which may cause you to break out into loud tears.

2. Mournful sorrow, during which you cry quietly, shedding many tears.

3. Depressive sorrow, in which you may not shed tears but show sorrow in your face.

4. Anger type of depression, in which you may want to cry but lack tears and are unable to make a sound. Sorrow embodies anger, and anger embodies sorrow.

Necessary Nutrients

Foods that can support us during times of grief include green and orange foods such as violet leaf, dandelion, kale, collards, carrots, winter squashes, and sweet potatoes, as they support the lungs and large intestines, which can become more vulnerable when you are grief stricken. Celery helps comfort the pangs of a broken heart. Use pungent condiments such as clove, coriander, and ginger to move lung stagnation.

Craving carbohydrates during periods of grief may be the body's attempt to elevate serotonin levels. Instead, try the supplement **5-HTP**, which helps your body make its own serotonin. **GABA** can help relieve cravings, including wanting a person who cannot be in your life the way you would like. The amino acid **tyrosine** will help elevate your mood by increasing dopamine levels.

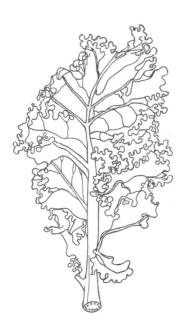

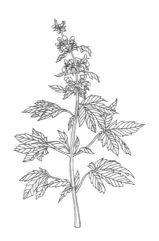

Healing Herbs for Grief

Herbs can be a great comforter during times of grief. Consider the benefits of hops, lemon balm, and passionflower. Saint-John's-wort is good to use when you are worn out from sobbing, while motherwort is a soothing remedy for grief. Try this formula for heartbreak-type sorrow: two parts hawthorn, one part motherwort, two parts lemon balm, and one part violet.

Well-Being Supplements

Vitamin B complex is a great ally during times of emotional distress.

Natural Practices

Homeopathic remedies that can be used for grief are:

Causticum: May be of benefit if you cry frequently or are experiencing forgetfulness and mental dullness.

Ignatia: For grief, loss, and hysteria, or if you sigh and can't sleep. You may be nervous and shake. You strongly identify with the person lost and feel you cannot exist without them. Use for disappointment in love or death.

Natrum muriaticum: When you dwell on the past, hold grudges, and reject sympathy. For death and loss of a loved one. When you have not been the same, are becoming withdrawn, not living life to the fullest.

Pulsatilla: When you are sad, yielding, indecisive, and weepy. You need to be with other people. Use for anxiety following bad news. For women who can't leave a bad relationship.

Use Flower Power

Some flower essences that are helpful include:

Bleeding heart: For grief related to the loss of a loved one or a separation. It helps to foster peace and detachment.

Borage: Use when you are discouraged during times of grief. Helps to lift your spirits. Gives you courage.

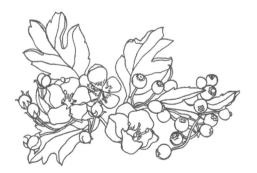

Hawthorn: Gives protection during periods of intense grief and stress.

Honeysuckle: Use when there is no adjustment months after the loss of a loved one. You are living in the past.

Mustard: For deep gloom that comes on strong then suddenly leaves. You may cry without knowing why.

Pear: For extreme grief, emergency situations that throw us off balance.

Star of Bethlehem: For great physical shock and trauma such as rape, injury, robbery, and accidents. It can also be used when you are having a difficult time coping with death of a pet or loved one. Edward Bach called this one "the comforter and soother of pains and sorrows."

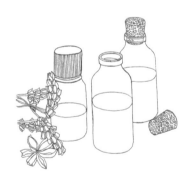

Aromatherapy Aid for Grief

Soaking in the bathtub can be a good place to let the tears flow. Add some essential oils such as cedarwood, clary sage, cypress, fir, frankincense, geranium, ginger, grapefruit, helichrysum, hyssop, lavender, jasmine, marjoram, neroli, orange, patchouli, rose, rosemary, rosewood, sage, sandalwood, spikenard, tangerine, or ylang-ylang. Melissa oil is good for heartbreak over a love relationship. All are dispellers of grief.

When you're done bathing, let the water out and visualize sorrow and sadness going down the drain and being healed by the earth as you stay in the tub. Afterward, massage diluted essential oil (8 ounces [235 ml] sunflower oil with 30 drops essential oil) over the heart and lungs after the bath. Or use the oils in a diffuser, or simply take up to ten deep inhalations directly from the bottle.

Get It Out/Let It Go

It is healthier to express grief than to suppress it. The force of grief is contractive, and expressing it and crying help to clear repression. After crying, asthma, hives, and muscular tension may disappear; blood pressure, pulse rate, and body temperature may lower; and more synchronized brain wave patterns may occur.

The Cleansing and Healing Power of Tears

Tears of emotional release are found to be higher in protein than tears caused by cutting onions. Emotional tears also include endorphin, which helps relieve pain, and the stress hormones norepinephrine and ACTH. Crying helps remove these chemical buildups.

If You Have Trouble Crying

If the tears won't come and you feel they might help heal your grief, there is a technique that can help. First you must create a safe space where you will not be disturbed. If others might hear you, give them advance notice to allow you your process without intervention.

Hold on to something such as a big teddy bear or body pillow. Place one hand on your collarbone. Start breathing only as deep as your hand. Then breathe more rapidly and make a sound. Hear the feelings in your voice and go ahead and sound like a crying baby.

Give yourself the space to feel the sadness. Think about what is causing it and let the tears flow. Accept the reality that the worst has happened. Gently lean into the pain. Stay with it. You'll find that it's not endless.

Let It Out

Groaning is also a method you can use to help dissipate sadness and pain. While groaning, think of the reasons for your suffering. When you exhale, visualize sorrow being exhaled from your being.

Let the Sun Shine

You can also release grief by standing facing the rising sun and letting its rays beam on your heart. Visualize the sun healing your grief while you breathe deeply, and the sorrow leaving your heart with each exhale.

Surviving a Breakup

A breakup can feel like a death. But when someone breaks up with you, do your best to stay calm. Screaming and throwing things tends to make the one departing feel justified that they made the right decision! When things simmer down in a few days, ask for their reasons for breaking up and make sure to review your own.

When you feel ready, put your ex's belongings into a box and return things with a minimum of drama. Be fair about giving back heirlooms and expensive things that were not gifts. It is not worth fighting over CDs or books, which can easily be replaced. Put mementos you wish to keep in a safe place.

Take some time before you get involved with someone again. Right after a breakup, you are apt to be especially vulnerable, and a period of time to yourself allows you to heal and regain your balance and independence. Allow sufficient time for mourning and healing before beginning another relationship, so you'll be less likely to project unresolved issues from your last partner onto your new one. The more intense the breakup, the more time you may need.

Next time you run into your ex, let them see the new, improved version! If they are with a new love, walk over and introduce yourself, making it sweet but brief. Show you have class! If you see them at a party and you are both alone, say hello, but refrain from leaving and having sex with them. Continuing to sleep with someone when the relationship is really over prolongs pain.

What NOT to Do after a Breakup

- Listen to the same music as you did when you were together.
- Hang out where you hope you will run into him or her.
- Call or run to your ex-partner when you are sad, scared, or depressed.
- Call just to check in.
- Sit and wait by the phone.
- Wallow in nostalgic thoughts about your ex; if you do, just say, "Eject."
- Overshop and spend.

What to Do:

- If you need help adjusting, make an appointment with a therapist or spiritual advisor.
- Get busy.
- Change your routine.
- Realize that now you get to be in charge of your life. Make your dreams come true!
- Improve the way you look.
- Get healthy.
- Exercise. It helps lift depression.
- Quit bad habits. Overdoing alcohol, drugs, and junk food will only make this time more difficult.
- Do your best to have no contact for at least thirty days—no calls, texting, or meeting up. Or you will backslide.

Closure Rituals

Sometimes things end so that we have an opportunity to evolve. Whether grief is due to death of a person or a relationship, you may want to have a closing ritual.

Create an altar by placing a photo of your departed, a sprig of rosemary (for remembrance), and a calming blue candle in a bowl filled with sand or dirt. Anoint the candle with a fragrance that reminds you of them, and etch their name into the candle.

Light the candle with a prayer of thanks for the lessons learned in the relationship, and as it burns down and out, reflect or write in your journal about the relationship. You can even play a song that reminds you of the person. Or consider a ritual such as writing a letter to get all of your feelings out and burning it in the fireplace, make a toast to a departed loved one, or light candles on important dates such as their birthday or your anniversary

Advice for Healing Grief of All Kinds

- As you heal, it's important to take care of yourself and indulge in pampering. Get plenty of rest and enjoy massages if possible. Connect with nature and take walks.
- Practice deep, slow breathing to cleanse emotions of grief. Exercise can also raise dopamine levels.
- The loving support of friends and family members can be a blessing. Call a few of your best friends over and allow them to cheer you up. Seek out those who want to see you happy and avoid negative people.
- It helps to have order in your life when you feel out of control. Clean up and clear out your house. Use feng shui to make it harmonious. Burn some sage or artemisia to clear away toxic emotions.
- Learn to be self-sufficient, love yourself and your own company, and you will attract the right people.
- Find a grief support group.
- When you feel better, and if you can, consider traveling to someplace new. Travel can help the heart and give you new perspectives. Read *Eat, Pray, Love* to inspire you.
- Wear and visualize the color violet to help heal grief.
- Wear rose quartz. Sleep with it in your hand and your dreams may have a healing effect upon your heart.
- Put energy into your career. Develop talents and work on your personal growth. Take a class. Read self-help books. Learn a new language.
- Ask God for help.

Let the Passage of Time Heal You

Time is a great healer. You will heal, and it helps to make a conscious decision to do so. Remember that setbacks are part of the process. You may feel that you have healed and then have another bad day where the pain is as intense as ever. This is normal and a sign that healing is happening. You are letting go of the past to make room for something new!

Journal Topic

When I went through a divorce, my massage therapist suggested I make a list of 100 reasons why it was better not to be with my partner. At first it was difficult and I could only come up with a few reasons, such as more time to myself and not having to make fancy dinners. Over time the list grew to well over 100 reasons, and I found this to be a powerful healing technique. Putting it on paper helped to get it out of me. It will help you, too.

If death or loss of love is the reason for grief, it can be very therapeutic to write about it:

- Start with how you met, what your feelings and expectations were.
- Write about memorable dates and events.
- Write about how each of you benefited one another.
- Make a list of what you have learned.
- Write down what you miss about them and perhaps even what bothered you about them.
- Give your story a title.

Remember that the pain of grief lessens over time. Total healing does not happen all at once, but past hurts can be healed at any time of life.

Releasing Trauma

"Crisis doesn't build character, it reveals it."
—Anonymous

Recovering from trauma, such as grief, is a process that takes time. Trauma can make you feel unsafe in your own body and with others. Trauma can be stored in the tissues. Body workers often say, "The issue is in the tissue."

 Good to Know!

The loving support of friends can be a great blessing. When a friend is grieving, "venture, validate, and volunteer." Ask your friend how they are doing, validate what they are saying, and volunteer to help in practical ways like taking them out to eat, babysitting, giving them a ride, etc. Acknowledge the person's suffering and listen to them.

Trauma can be verbal, physical, psychological, sexual, and/or violent. Rape, miscarriage, kidnapping, earthquake, fire, robbery, violent attacks, war, plane crash, mass destruction, surgery, difficult birth, and abortion to mention just a few, are all examples of trauma.

The Aftereffects of Trauma

If you've been traumatized, you may be unable to let go of the anxiety associated with the experience, remaining overwhelmed and terrified. Panic attacks, anxiety, flashbacks, rage, repetitive destructive behaviors, being emotionally closed, depression, and insomnia may follow traumatic episodes.

The traumatic experience may be blocked but not erased, continuing to exist as an electrical chemical energy locked in the brain, exerting a force that can contribute to nervousness, irritation, or depression. If trauma is not acknowledged and dealt with, it can continue to affect your life and relationships.

Good to Know!

In tribal society, a healing ceremony is held for the traumatized person. With the help of community, the person is assisted in reuniting with their lost spirit. After being cleansed with smoke, sound, and herbs, a medicine man or woman may call the person's spirit back into their body, and a joyous celebration welcomes them back.

Ask for Positive Support

Having the support of family and friends can be a great ally in any sort of trauma. Thank them for feeling safe and sharing their soul and feelings with you.

Offer encouragement such as "It's okay. I'm here for you. I care." Avoid correcting or analyzing. Offer support by saying, "I'm glad you told me." Things not to say include "Get over it. Put it behind you. I know something that happened to so and so and she became an Olympic athlete," or "Oh, you poor thing."

When it comes to you, expressing feelings of grief, anger (see sections on grief and anger in this chapter), and hurt may be difficult but can help you release old stored emotions, and move on.

Skip This!

Avoid caffeine and sugar, which will stress your already compromised nervous system. See chapters 2 and 3 for more healing solutions.

Necessary Nutrients

Choose comforting foods after trauma. Eat warm, nourishing foods such as soups. Or ask a friend to make up your favorite healthy dish.

Healing Herbs

Soothe the aftereffects of trauma with oatstraw, motherwort, raspberry leaf tea, Saint-John's-wort, schizandra berries, and eleuthero. All are nerve-nourishing tonics that can help you heal.

Well-Being Supplements

Try **7-keto DHEA** to help relieve moods and symptoms associated with post-traumatic stress.

Use **a Chinese patent formula** for post-traumatic stress, bad fright, or severe shock to the emotional body. It's called **Ding Xin Wan**, also known as **Calm Heart Pill**.

Homeopathic arnica can help heal trauma.

Natural Practices for Healing

Aromatherapy. Taking up to deep ten inhalations of essential oil of lavender from the bottle will help calm and relax you. Rose essential oil helps soothe emotional traumas. Take an aromatherapy bath, using a pound (455 g) of sea salt and seven drops of lavender essential oil or rose oil.

Flower essences. Rescue Remedy is the Bach Flower Remedy for panic, shock, grief, despair, and other crisis. Take two drops under the tongue to help you find your center again.

More flower essences for trauma:

Hibiscus: For women who have been sexually traumatized.

Mariposa lily: Helps alleviate trauma from sexual abuse as a child.

Star of Bethlehem: For great physical shock and trauma such as rape, injury, robbery, and serious accidents.

Soak your feet in warm water to which a half teaspoon of cayenne pepper has been added and stirred.

Surround yourself with the healing color green. Green clothes, green bedding, green foods, and have green plants in your midst.

Breathe in love, breathe out, and cleanse yourself of hurt feelings.

Call on God, Great Spirit, higher powers, and/ or angels, or whatever your personal beliefs include for the healing.

Holistic Therapies for Healing

Acupressure. Apply pressure to the point two-thirds up from upper lip to nose.

Use the power of a shower. Use a pulsing showerhead to help overcome the numbness sometimes associated with trauma after physical healing is under way. Take slow sessions, directing the spray on various regions of the body, head, face, and feet, being sure to include every part.

Be present with each part, using water that is a comfortable temperature, and remind yourself, "This is my chest, this is my back. I welcome you back." Gently doing self-massage or gentle tapping can also be of benefit. Be patient and gentle with the healing process.

Volunteer work can help undo the past, by helping others in a similar situation. Be proactive. If rape has occurred, take a self-defense class to be more empowered.

Journal Topic

Help heal your wounds by writing about your feelings rather than repeating the story over and over and reliving the past. Once you've written your feelings down, you can give it to a trusted friend to read, and once she has, discuss it.

For more exercises on overcoming trauma read *Waking the Tiger* by Peter A. Levine.

Dealing with Angry Feelings

Anger is part of the grieving process (which is known by the acronym DABDA: Denial, Anger,

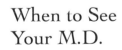

When to See Your M.D.

To heal, don't try to go it alone. Professional counseling and medication can help you recover, even if the trauma occurred years ago. Honesty, awareness, communication, and commitment are essential for healing.

Think about This...

Anger can be beneficial if it contributes to change. For example, if people had not gotten angry, women would still not be able to vote and people of color would still not have the rights they are entitled to.

Bargaining, Depression, and Acceptance) and recovering from trauma, and it's also a very common emotion in everyday life. We can become angry when our desire for something or someone meets resistance, and when we don't get what we want, whether it is love, happiness, recognition, reward, justice, money, ease, fame, or respect.

Studies show that people who are overly disruptive and behave aggressively often have low levels of serotonin, the feel-good hormone that helps transmit nerve impulses from one neuron to another.

Anger: The Traditional Chinese Medicine Perspective

In Traditional Chinese Medicine, anger is seen as a hot emotion of ascending chi or Liver Yang Rising. The emotion of anger correlates to the liver. An unhealthy liver may aggravate anger, and excess anger can injure the liver. Interestingly, the word *bilious* refers to bad temper as well as liver problems. The goal in clearing anger is to correct the cause, reduce heat, and move stagnation.

The Effect of Anger on Your Body

The hormones catecholamine, adrenaline, and noradrenaline rev you up for immediate action. But adrenaline does not become an "anger hormone" until you are provoked, or you interpret events in a negative way.

Anger has an extreme effect on your body. It causes shallow inhalation and strong, panting exhalation, dizziness, high blood pressure, increased circulation, elevated cholesterol levels, tight shoulders, stiff upper back, jaw tightness, eye problems, increased hydrochloric acid production, and ulcers.

Clumsiness, irritability, and impatience are also characteristics of anger. Procrastination, accidentally destroying the "enemy's" property, and losing items may also be anger symptoms surfacing. Anger and violence are also linked to low blood sugar (hypoglycemia) as well as fear, anxiety, panic, and fatigue.

Some people describe anger as making them "see red." Exposure to heavy metals such as lead can also contribute to delinquent and angry behavior.

Holding Anger In

Expressing anger in a safe way is healthier than repressing it. Pent-up angry feelings can be a factor in hemorrhoids, migraine headaches, cancer, rheumatoid arthritis, and heart disease. Years of anger can block blood flow to the coronary artery. It's important that anger is released in a natural, gentle way, never on other people, pets, or any living thing. Try going past a train track and screaming as the train rushes by or punching a pillow, using a punching bag, or using a foam bat to beat up tough furniture.

Necessary Nutrients

Foods that benefit the liver and mellow the emotion of anger include artichokes, barley, daikon radish, green leafy vegetables (especially dandelion greens), lemon, lentils, mung beans, rye, sour green apples, and white beans. Dandelion root helps to cleanse emotions of anger stored in the liver.

Healing Herbs

Herbs that help cool the liver and thus soothe anger include blessed thistle, bupleurum, dandelion root, dong quai, licorice root, oatstraw, passionflower, peony root, and skullcap.

Skip This!

Excess garlic, onions, and coffee can be too hot and aggravate anger and make you more likely to fly off the handle.

Well-Being Supplements

Supplements that can help ease an angry countenance include B complex and 5-HTP (5-hydroxtryptophan), an amino acid. 5-HTP is derived from the *Griffonia simplicifolia* plant in the Fabaceae family found in West Africa that along with behavior counseling can help correct neurotransmitter imbalance and curb anger.

In addition, taking a multi-amino-acid formula that contains phenylalanine, leucine, valine, histidine, arginine, lysine, isoleucine, alanine, glutamine, methionine, and threonine can help ice anger, along with GTF chromium and calcium with magnesium. The DHA in fish oil can also help.

Natural Practices to Soothe Anger Away

Homeopathic remedies that can cool fire in the liver include:

Chamomilla: For angry children or those constantly discontent.

Lachesis: For outbursts and irrational jealousy or when you are domineering, vicious, suspicious, and talkative.

Lycopodium: For the insecure person who takes anger out on others.

Mercuris: For sudden anger with an impulse to do violence. You are restless, agitated, or have poor memory, lack of concentration, or rapid speech. You are aggravated by many environmental influences and comfortable in few conditions.

Natrum muriaticum: For when you are unable to express anger.

Nux vomica: For those who have a possible violent temper and destructive impulses. You are fussy and fastidious over small things and dislike being contraindicated. You are hurried, impatient, and overemphasize achievement. You're a workaholic, annoyed by noise, persnickety, or domineering and can have a violent temper. You often have digestive disorders.

Sepia: For those who are critical of partners, argumentative, and pessimistic.

Staphysagria: For helping ailments caused by repressed anger. Benefits those that hold their temper until they blow up.

Sulfur: For the know-it-all person who is haughty yet philosophical, creative, and impractical or who argues for the entertainment of it.

Flower essences that assist in calming anger include:

Cherry plum: For when you feel you are about to do something desperate and for those prone to temper tantrums.

Heather: For those who are easily irritated.

Holly: For helping with jealousy and sibling rivalry.

Impatiens: For people who feel irritable and impatient.

Walnut: For protection from outside influences that cause anger. Also helps one going through big life changes.

Aromatherapy Aid

Essential oils that can be used as aromatherapy include basil, cardamom, chamomile, champa, coriander, frankincense, geranium, hyssop, jasmine, lavender, lemon balm (melissa), lotus, marjoram, neroli, patchouli, pine, rose, rosewood, and ylang-ylang. Use them in a diffuser, inhale five to ten times from the bottle, or use them in a nice, warm bath. Soak your anger away!

Bodywork, like massage, can help to soften the liver and soothe a savage spirit. Yoga helps by improving flexibility in body and mind. A calming folk remedy is to get buried in the sand, with your face uncovered, of course!

Advice for Easing and Letting Go of Anger

Try to Relax

- As soon as you feel angry, focus on breathing deeply. Affirm that you are angry.
- Try counting to ten while visualizing the calming color blue. There may be some occasions where you need to count to one hundred! Drink some cold water.

Express How You Feel Clearly

- Be clear about what is really bothering you. If necessary, remove yourself from a hot situation and return when you can more safely express yourself.
- If you write an angry letter or vent your anger before your heart rate has calmed down, you may regret it, so collect your thoughts first and then express them. Clear, respectful, and nonaggressive language works best.

- Consider humor a more valuable ally than profanity. Without attacking, let your feelings be known.

What to Do

- Make eye contact with the person you are arguing with.
- Listen to what the other person has to say without interrupting and do your best to understand. Nod or say "yes" to indicate you are listening. Mirror back what they say. Be willing to forgive!
- Use your anger to get creative. One of my teachers, Michael Tierra, would say, "Art is toxic discharge." So get out there and paint, write, create music, or find some way to express yourself and contribute to your own therapy.
- Learn what triggers your anger and try to avoid those situations.

What Not to Do

- Use profanity and scream at the other person. It can impair your ability to be heard.
- Use statements such as "you always" or "you never." Stick with the issue at hand.
- Resort to name-calling and blaming, going for the jugular, and threats either physical or verbal.
- Use a hostile expression. It can aggravate emotions, resolve nothing, and even put you and others in peril. Avoid pointing fingers or using defensive language such as crossing your arms in front of you.

Journal Topic

To put things into perspective, write up a disaster scale and rate the things that make you angry from one to ten, with ten being the highest. You may find that some of them are not as important as you thought they were!

Make a list about what aspects of the anger you are accountable for. Write about what you can do about it. Make amends if you can. Be kind to yourself and others.

Recovering from Addiction

If you have trouble with addiction, you can leave it behind, along with grief, trauma, and anger. Inner craving for deep spiritual connection, stress, anxiety, genetics, cultural factors, nutritional deficiencies, allergies, and neurotransmitter imbalances are often at the roots of addiction. Addiction can bring on psychological and emotional problems or it can be the result of them.

All mood-altering activities tend to initially produce a sense of euphoria. The posteuphoric stage is followed by a low, which causes the person to seek another episode of repeating the activity.

Joining one of the many twelve-step support groups can help, along with getting counseling or therapy, working with your doctor and other trained mental health professionals. In addition, try these natural cures to help you recover from addiction.

Good to Know!

There may be a correlation between addiction and blood sugar problems. Support groups for addicts often provide coffee and cookies. It may be wise to cut back or give up sugar if you have addictive tendencies. Check out *Beat Sugar Addiction Now!* for more information.

Necessary Nutrients

When recovering from addiction, focus on cleansing, rebuilding, and nurturing yourself. Get more alkaline by consuming more fresh fruits and vegetables. Use foods that help the liver clean itself out such as apples, artichokes, beets, burdock root, carrots, celery, daikon radish, green leafy vegetables, persimmons, and hemp seed oil. Drink the juice of one half lemon in water several times daily to detoxify the liver.

Sea vegetables help nourish the thyroid gland and endocrine system. Superfoods such as blue-green algae, spirulina, and chlorella can be highly nutritive and rebuilding for the person giving up an addiction of any sort.

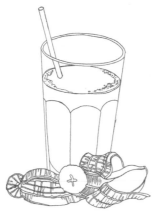

A **Super-Tonic Smoothie** can be nutritive and energizing. Here's how to make one—just blend the following ingredients:

> 1 cup (235 ml) almond milk
> Half a ripe banana
> 1/2 teaspoon ginseng powder
> 1 teaspoon spirulina powder
> 1 tablespoon (16 g) raw almond butter
> 1 tablespoon (8 g) nutritional yeast

 ## Healing Herbs

Herbs that can help overcome addiction include:

Basil leaf is a nerve restorative that lifts the spirits from depression and calms anxiety.

Cinnamon bark improves circulation and is stimulating yet calming to the nerves. Cinnamon is naturally sweet, thereby satisfying the body's desires for other substances.

Clove bud helps reduce cravings and is a natural antioxidant, expectorant, and stimulant.

Dandelion root helps detoxify the body, cleansing the liver and stimulating digestion.

Fennel seed is naturally sweet, which helps stabilize blood sugar levels and thereby decrease the desire for substances while improving energy levels.

Lemon balm leaf helps during withdrawal and detox periods by lifting the spirits and supporting the nervous system.

Milk thistle seed can be used to help rebuild a damaged liver.

Oatstraw herb calms and strengthens the nerves, lessens anxiety, and decreases the desire for substances.

Saint-John's-wort helps relieve depression and anxiety that cause you to turn to addictive substances for temporary relief.

Skullcap calms the emotions, enhances awareness, and quiets overexcitability. It also helps curb the emotional need and cravings for addictive substances.

Note: If alcohol is the addiction, use herbs as tea, glycerites, or capsules rather than in alcohol tincture form.

 ## Well-Being Supplements

When giving up an addiction, nurture yourself with some good vitamin-mineral supplements. Vitamin C is detoxifying and can reduce cravings. A calcium-magnesium supplement is especially helpful in giving the nervous system support and promoting calmness when giving up an addiction. The B complex helps diminish withdrawal symptoms and aids liver regeneration. A supplement of GTF (glucose tolerance factor) chromium helps to regulate blood sugar levels and metabolize carbohydrates.

Natural Practices
Aromatherapy

Essential oils can be most helpful in giving up an addiction. Every time you crave an addictive substance, take deep inhalations of essential oils of basil, cardamom, fennel, and/or rosemary. Soak in a bathtub to which 3 pounds (1.4 kg) of Epsom salts and 8 to 10 drops of essential oils have been added to relax and detox your system.

Sauna baths can also speed up the release of toxic substances. The sooner you can get it out of your system, the easier it will be to let go of it.

Breathe! Deep breathing is calming as well as energizing and provides our brains with a much-needed substance: oxygen. Exercise also increases the amount of oxygen available to the body.

Holistic Practices

Acupuncture has helped many people overcome addictions because of its ability to stimulate detoxification and encourage endorphin production.

More Ways to Leave Addiction Behind

Decide to change. Refuse to be enslaved by anything. Learn to deal with any lapses in a positive, healing way. Be a free, conscious being.

Find new, more productive ways of acting. For example, compulsive spenders may need to purchase only those items that they can buy with cash or a check.

Make a list of positive ways to reward yourself. For example, instead of having coffee every morning, go for a walk. Instead of a drink at night, take an aromatherapy bath or make a phone call to a friend.

Take up some new activities or a craft. This can be a help to improve your self-esteem.

Write down on a note card all the reasons to give up the addiction. When tempted to backslide, pull the card out and reread the reasons.

Draw a picture of your addiction to help you gain perspective. For example, a monkey on your back.

Good to Know!

If you feel the urge to backslide, call a drug-free friend. Warn friends that you may be grumpy and give them some suggestions on how they can be supportive to you. Ask former addicts to tell you how giving up the addiction has benefited them. Initially, it is wise to avoid the places where you know your addiction will be indulged in.

Have someone photograph you indulging in your addiction while you look into the camera. When you get the photo back, look at it carefully and ask yourself what it is trying to tell you. Put all that extra energy into doing something good, something that helps both society and yourself.

Try writing to your addiction with your right hand, describing how it affects you. Now with your left hand, have your addiction "write back to you." This can help reveal some of your inner-child behavior.

Use color. The color blue helps you to relax and cools inflammation. Green is balancing. Wear or surround yourself with these colors when you can.

Be consistent and keep track of your progress, such as posting it on the refrigerator. Consider showing the progress chart to someone you really trust. Tell them you are not asking them to nag at you, but tell them in what ways they can best help you.

Do what it takes to have a clean, uncluttered place so your consciousness will not be encumbered. A planner either on paper or on your phone can help your mind feel more organized so that life will feel less stressful.

Change your reward system. Instead of choosing addictive substances, save the money that you would have spent. Use the money for things to improve your life—books, clothes, a vacation.

Find ways to nurture yourself. Good nutrition, massage, biofeedback, hypnotism, exercise, meditation, and prayer may all be healing on deep levels. Find ways to reward yourself each day—for example, a massage, a foot rub, and a long-distance phone call to a favorite friend.

Fulfill your true spiritual quest. What do you believe in? What matters most? Find out and then do something about it!

Journal topic: Make a list of the reasons why you should stop. Put it where you can often read it—above a sink, on a mirror, on a bookmark, in your wallet. Being clear about why you want to give up a habit is very important.

Wise Advice from Brigitte on Addiction

Addiction keeps us stuck and impairs our ability to grow. So stop postponing. This is the moment! You deserve to be happy and free. The first step is to admit there is a problem. The second step is to do something about it.

Best wishes to all of you who are brave enough to let go of that which does not benefit your life!

For more info on overcoming addictions, check out my book *Addiction-Free Naturally*.

Chapter 12

CULTIVATE JOY AND HAPPINESS

A merry heart doeth like a medicine and a broken spirit dryeth the bone.

—Proverbs 17:22

Both happiness and joy contribute to good health, so they are worth learning more about, cultivating, and enjoying. Speaking of joy, this emotion balances the function of the cardiac system and excites the cerebral cortex and the autonomic and sympathetic nervous systems. Joy eases the flow of chi, helping us to relax and feel more harmonious. Happiness increases the activity of the internal organs and rate of digestive secretions.

Mother Nature's News
(Yoga) Laughter *Is* the Best Medicine!

Laughter elevates the levels of feel-good brain chemicals like endorphins that make you feel more positive and happy. Laughter also shakes and caresses the heart, causing it to let go of stored tensions; dilates blood vessels; improves circulation; increases oxygen intake; and boosts immune health. After a session of laughter, breathing and heart rate slow, blood pressure drops, and muscles relax.

Now there is a yoga practice that encourages jocularity to improve health: laughter yoga. More and more people are practicing yoga laughter each day, and it is now widely used in hospitals to speed healing and to help ease depression in chronically ill patients.

In 2006, Laughter Yoga International commissioned a research project to study laughter yoga's effects on stress levels in IT professionals in Bangalore, India. Half of the group attended seven laughter yoga sessions over an eighteen-day period. The results proved that laughter is the best medicine. The laughter yoga group experienced a significant drop in heart rate, blood pressure, and stress hormones. Laughter yoga also helps promote a positive state of mind. In this study, glass half full or positive emotions increased by 17 percent and glass half empty or negative emotions dropped by 27 percent. Visit www.laughteryoga.org to join the fun and get healthy!

Good to Know!

According to the principles of Asian medicine, the Heart/Fire System is said to correspond to the emotion of joy, as well as lack of joy. The Fire Element corresponds to laughter and the spirit, provides energy for circulation, and is often described as "the emperor, ruling all the other organs."

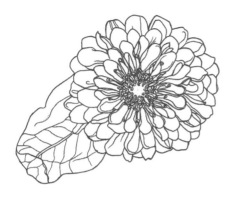

Flower Power

If you have a hard time laughing, the flower essence zinnia (*Zinnia elegans*) can help foster lightness, humor, and release of tension. It can also help you delight in life's joy and inner-child wonder.

What TCM Says

According to Traditional Chinese Medicine, an imbalance in the Heart or Fire Element interferes with joy and can manifest itself as a racing heart, speech problems, and sweating easily.

If you have problems with your Fire Element, eat more bitter foods such as dandelion leaves and kale and drink reishi mushroom and green tea. Add more colorful fresh fruits and vegetables in season to make life more joyous by flooding your body with both antioxidants and phytonutrients.

Joyful, happy people are said to live longer. These tips, ideas, and strategies will help you see the sunny side of life more of the time, improving your life, health, and well-being.

1. Turn your problems over to a Higher Power. Having a spiritual path feeds the soul and keeps you connected to the divine plan of the universe.

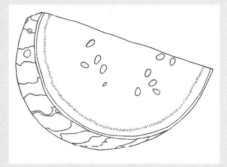

2. When difficulties occur, sit by a river and let go, and go with the flow. Accept and move on. Look for the positive things that can happen from a negative experience.

3. Getting all the facts can help you accept the situation, so gather data. Ask others to share some insight on the situation.

4. Instead of brooding over things gone wrong, review the event, then fully experience your feelings for one minute and turn your attention to something else. Repeat as often as necessary.

5. Accept the current reality. Choose to create what you want in life. Take action to create what you want. Focus on the experience you want to have.

6. "He who laughs, lasts." Bring more humor into your life. Read the comics. Watch comedies. Ask others if they know any good jokes. Learn some yourself!

7. Associate with positive people. Avoid negative influences and people that drag you down. Connect with inspiring people.

8. Share life and joy with loved ones. Spending time with children and having loving relationships can increase quality of life.

9. Adopt a rescue dog or cat. People that have pets are likely to live longer and enjoy more disease-free and happy lives.

10. Let go of trying to please everyone. Avoid taking things personally. Look for the similarities in one another and don't get hung up on the differences.

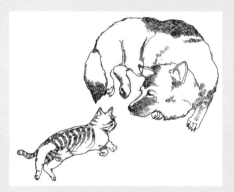

11. Communicate your feelings. Those that withdraw are more prone to cancer and suicide. Those that are angry and hostile are more likely candidates for heart attacks. Optimists have fewer chronic diseases.

12. Instead of saying yes or no right away, you can say, "I'll think about it."

13. Help someone in need. Reach out and touch others. Volunteer.

14. Look for activities, many of which are free in your local paper. Often the library, bookstores, or concerts in the park provide great fun and an opportunity to learn something new as you mingle with others.

15. Clean out clutter. It contributes to feeling stuck and blocked. Get rid of things that no longer serve.

16. Rearrange your home. Learn about feng shui as a way to improve every area of your life.

17. Stop spending money on things that you don't need.

18. Make health a positive priority that includes good nutrition, meditation, and exercise. Do at least seven healthy things daily.

19. Spending time in Nature can help you develop inner peace. Get outdoors in full-spectrum light for at least a few minutes each day. Take a walk almost every day.

20. Have potlucks with friends. Inspire each other to try new foods and eat healthier.

21. Creative people tend to be more flexible and enjoy life more. Take up a craft, draw, sculpt, and paint. Making things of beauty improves self-esteem and can help relieve tension.

22. Keep learning your entire life.

23. Planting a garden shows belief in the future and brings joy and life lessons daily.

24. Spend your time reading books that are uplifting and watching shows that have value rather than filling your consciousness with violence and despair.

25. Let go of the past. Every experience in life has taught you something or made you stronger. You can choose to move on from past hurts.

26. Essential oils that promote feelings of joy include basil, bergamot, neroli, orange, and rose.

27. Flowers that help to calm the spirit and promote joy include roses, chrysanthemum, lotus, orchid, jasmine, and narcissus. They may help you lighten up.

28. Do your best to have a good life while you are here. Do something to make the world a little bit better for your having been here!

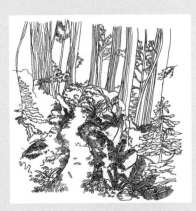

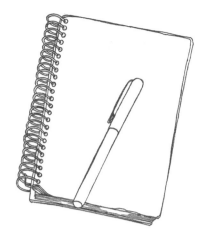

Journal Topics

- Make a list of the difficulties in your life. Go through the list and see which one of these things you can let go of.
- Write down what you need to do. Honor your commitments.
- Make a list of 100 things you want to accomplish in your life. Put a check by those you achieve. Update the list as you achieve your goals.
- Make a list of your past successes, awards, and accomplishments.
- Make a list of ten things you love. Make a list of ten things you are good at. Consider a career based on where some of those things intersect.
- Make a list of the things you truly are grateful for.

Thank you for beginning your journey to health, happiness, and well-being with me. With a little effort, you can make real and lasting changes in your life. Start on the path today by taking the first step!

Appendix A

ESSENTIAL HERBS

Numerous herbs benefit conditions of your mind, nervous system, and body. Here you'll find detailed information about the most commonly used herbs, contraindications, and instructions for use. If you have any questions, see your health care practitioner.

1. Ashwagandha

Withania somnifera
Solanaceae (nightshade) family

Medicinal Uses

Ashwagandha's use has been recorded for at least 3,000 years. It builds chi, helps lower cortisol levels, and is excellent for those in convalescence. Ashwagandha makes the body more resistant to stress and prevents depletion of vitamin C. It helps prevent stress-related ulcers. Ashwagandha nourishes and calms the mind, promotes sleep, and improves brain function in the elderly. Use it for anxiety, bipolar disorder, exhaustion, memory loss, mental fatigue, neuroses, overwork, panic attacks, and stress.

It works best over a prolonged period of time. An Ayurvedic maxim says that taking ashwagandha for fifteen days imparts strength to the emaciated body, just as rain does to a crop.

Contraindications

During pregnancy use ashwagandha only under the guidance of a health care professional, because there have been reports of the herb having abortifacient properties. Using this herb in combination with barbiturates can exacerbate their effects. The berries have caused gastrointestinal distress when consumed by children. Do not use the leaf in cases of congestion.

2. Astragalus

Astragalus hoangtchy, A. membranaceus, A. mongolicus (syn. *A. propinquus*)
Fabaceae (pea) family

Medicinal Uses

Astragalus is one of the most widely prescribed herbs in Chinese medicine. Generally it is used not to treat any disease in particular but to enhance and balance bodily functions.

Astragalus helps increase vitality, builds the blood, normalizes the hormones, and improves circulation. It bolsters the wei chi, or the defensive immune system. It eases worry.

Contraindications

Astragalus is not recommended in cases of severe congestion, extreme tension, or an overactive immune system. It is generally not recommended in cases of fever and inflammation or extreme dryness (as evidenced by persistent thirst, dry skin, and constipation). It is best to avoid its use in cases of hot, toxic skin lesions and at the onset of cold and flu symptoms. It tends to hold infection in the body, so if you use astragalus during cases of infection, combine it with diaphoretic herbs.

Wild North American astragalus, often called locoweed, should not be used until further research has been done, since it may contain in its leaves toxic alkaloids that contribute to heart and lung suppression. Livestock that have consumed locoweed have been known to jump over imaginary objects, wander aimlessly, and drool excessively.

3. Black Cohosh

Actaea racemosa (formerly *Cimicifuga racemosa*)
Ranunculaceae (buttercup) family

Medicinal Uses
Black cohosh improves circulation and lowers blood pressure. It helps emotional instability, hysteria, mania, melancholy, moodiness, stress, and anxiety related to menopause. It is a nerve sedative because of its potassium and magnesium content.

As a flower essence, black cohosh helps those who are in abusive and addictive relationships. It aids you in building up the courage to confront rather than retreat and to transform the negative; it helps balance negative situations.

Contraindications
Avoid during pregnancy and while nursing, except under the guidance of a qualified health care practitioner. Avoid also in cases of heart conditions. Excess use can irritate the nervous system and cause nausea, vomiting, headache, and low blood pressure.

Unlike pharmaceutical hormone replacement therapy, black cohosh is considered to be a menopause tonic that is safe for women with estrogen-dependent cancers, uterine bleeding, fibrocystic breast disease, endometriosis, liver disease, gallbladder disease, or pancreatitis. Recently concern has arisen regarding the effect of this herb on the liver over the long term; further research is under way to investigate this issue.

Black cohosh is at risk of becoming endangered in the wild, so instead of wild crafting, consider cultivating your own supplies. When purchasing black cohosh products, be sure they are made only from cultivated stock.

4. Borage

Borago officinalis
Boraginaceae (borage) family

Medicinal Uses
Borage leaves, flowers, and seed oil moisten yin and clear heat. They help you feel happier and inspire courage. Borage helps relieve anxiety, grief, heartbreak, and worry.

The leaves and flowers have long been used in treatments for convalescence, depression, fevers, grief, hypertension, and worry.

As a flower essence, borage is used to lighten depression and discouragement. It helps bring joy, optimism, enthusiasm, and good cheer, improves confidence and courage, and dispels sadness in the face of danger and troubles.

Other Uses

In 1597, herbalist John Gerard quoted in his writings an old saying, "Ego borago gaudia semper ago," meaning "I, borage, always bring courage." In fact, the flowers have long been used to bolster courage (perhaps the fact that they nourish the adrenal glands explains why). In medieval times, the flowers were embroidered on the mantles of knights and jousters to give them courage, and they were also floated in drinks given to Crusaders as they took their leave. They were also sneaked into the drinks of prospective husbands to give them the courage to propose!

Contraindications

The leaf contains pyrrolizidine alkaloids, which are possibly toxic; use the leaf only in moderation unless further research negates the danger of these alkaloids. Avoid the leaf during pregnancy and while nursing.

5. Chamomile

Chamaemelum nobile (Roman chamomile; syn. *Anthemis nobilis*), *Matricaria recutita* (German chamomile; formerly *Chamomilla recutita*; syn. *M. chamomilla*)
Asteraceae (daisy) family

Medicinal Uses

Since the times of ancient Greece, both types of chamomile have been used medicinally in the same ways. It is a gentle relaxant that tones the nervous system and a nerve restorative for an exhausted system. It has traditionally been used to calm those prone to nightmares.

Chamomile is rich in the nerve and muscle nutrients calcium, magnesium, and potassium.

Chamomile moves chi, relaxes the nerves, reduces inflammation, clears toxins, and promotes sleep. Considered a nerve restorative, it calms anxiety and stress. It's a useful herb for those who are bothered by almost everything. Add chamomile tea to a child's bath before bed to help him or her sleep peacefully. It reduces whininess in children.

Chamomile is high in muscle-relaxing calcium, magnesium, potassium, and some of the B vitamins, which are known to aid relaxation. Chamomile is known for its anti-inflammatory and antispasmodic properties that can help a tense person unwind.

Contraindications

Some people, especially those who are sensitive to ragweed, may be severely allergic to chamomile. It can cause contact dermatitis in some individuals. Roman chamomile is more likely to cause an allergic reaction than the German variety. On the other hand, chamomile is sometimes used to treat allergies. Use the herb with caution the first time you try it. Otherwise, chamomile is considered very safe. Avoid therapeutic dosages during pregnancy.

6. Eleuthero

Eleuthero (*Eleutherococcus senticosus*, *E. gracilistylus*), formerly *Acanthopanax senticosus*, and *A. spinosus*
Araliaceae (ginseng) family

Medicinal Uses

Eleuthero has been used for centuries by the tribe peoples of Siberia and the Chinese. An ancient Chinese proverb is, "I would rather take a handful of eleuthero than a cartload of gold and jewels." In the frigid regions of China,

Russia, and Japan, reindeer, a symbol of strength and endurance, consume this plant.

Russian cosmonauts since 1962 have been given rations of eleuthero to help acclimate to the stresses of being weightless and living in space. Athletes, deep-sea divers, rescue workers, and explorers all use it for nourishment during times of stress. In the past forty years, more than 1,000 studies on eleuthero have shown that it shares many of the same therapeutic properties as Panax ginsengs.

Eleuthero nourishes the adrenals. It's considered an adaptogen and can help you acclimate to stressful situations. It improves endurance, moods, work productivity, and accuracy. It helps the body cope with stress. Use when exhausted, fatigued, and weak. Eleuthero is used to treat alcoholism, anxiety, chronic fatigue, and stress.

Contraindications

In rare cases, eleuthero may contribute to diarrhea, elevation of blood pressure, and mild blood-platelet antiaggregation properties. Taking eleuthero too close to bedtime may interfere with sleep.

7. Dandelion

Taraxacum officinale
Asteraceae (daisy) family

Medicinal Uses

Dandelion is one of the planet's most famous and useful weeds. This wonderful plant is a blood purifier that aids in the process of filtering and straining wastes from the bloodstream. It cools heat and clears infection from the body. It is especially useful in treating obstructions of the gallbladder, liver, pancreas, and spleen.

Dandelion is also used to help clear the body of old emotions such as anger and fear that can be stored in the liver and kidneys. Its leaves can be used to treat anorexia, appetite loss, bedwetting, breast cancer, candida, debility, fatigue, flatulence, hangover, high cholesterol, hypertension, hypochondria, insomnia, nervousness, and obesity.

The root is used primarily for liver-related problems. It is used to treat alcoholism, allergies, anorexia, appetite loss, candida, depression, dizziness, fatigue, hangover, headache, hypertension, hypochondria, hypoglycemia, obesity, osteoarthritis, ovarian cysts, and premenstrual syndrome.

As a flower essence, dandelion reduces tension, especially muscular tension in the neck, back, and shoulders. It fosters spiritual openness and encourages the letting go of fear and trust in one's own ability to cope with life. It can be beneficial for those who love life but tend to overextend themselves.

Contraindications

Dandelion is generally regarded as safe, even in large amounts and during pregnancy. However, as is the case with any plant, there is always a possibility of an allergic reaction. A few cases have been reported of abdominal discomfort, loose stools, nausea, and heartburn associated with dandelion. The fresh latex of the plant can cause contact dermatitis in sensitive individuals.

Consult with a qualified health care practitioner prior to using dandelion in cases of obstructed bile duct or gallstones. Individuals who have gastric hyperacidity may find that excessive use of dandelion leaf aggravates the condition.

8. Ginger

Zingiber officinale

Zingiberaceae (ginger) family

Medicinal Uses

Ginger has been found to be even more effective than Dramamine in curbing motion sickness, without causing drowsiness. As a digestive aid, it warms the digestive organs, stimulates digestive secretions, increases the amylase concentration in saliva, and facilitates the digestion of starches and fatty foods.

It also strengthens the tissues of the heart, activates the immune system, prevents blood platelet aggregation and leukotriene formation, and inhibits prostaglandin production, thus reducing inflammation and pain. Gingerroot is used in the treatment of anxiety, depression, fatigue, headache, hypertension, hypothyroidism, indigestion, obesity, and pain.

Topically, ginger can be prepared as a compress and applied over arthritic joints, bunions, sore muscles, and toothaches to relieve pain; over the kidneys to relieve the pain and assist in the passage of stones; over the chest or back to relieve asthma symptoms; or over the temples to relieve headache. Ginger is wonderful in the bath in cases of chills, muscle soreness, sciatica, and poor circulation.

Contraindications

Although ginger can relieve morning sickness, pregnant women should not ingest more than 1 gram daily. Avoid in cases of peptic ulcers, hyperacidity, or other hot, inflammatory conditions. Avoid excessive amounts of ginger in cases of acne, eczema, or herpes.

Ginger may cause adverse reactions when used in combination with anticoagulant drugs such as Coumadin or aspirin; if you are using such medications, seek the advice of a qualified health care practitioner before commencing use of ginger.

9. Ginkgo

Ginkgo biloba

Ginkgoaceae (ginkgo) family

Medicinal Uses

Ginkgo is the oldest tree species on the planet, having been common even when dinosaurs roamed the earth! It has a high resistance to disease, insects, and pollution.

It improves nerve transmission and helps the brain to better utilize oxygen and glucose. Ginkgo has been found to improve nerve signal transmission and activate ATP (adenosine triposphate), an organic compound that aids metabolic reactions. Ginkgo helps protect nerve cells from free-radical damage.

It is one of the best-selling medicines in Europe and used in the treatment of a wide variety of disorders associated with aging, including dementia, memory loss, and senility and to promote recovery from stroke. It is an antioxidant and cerebral tonic.

Ginkgo leaf enhances neurotransmitter receptor binding sites and neurotransmitter metabolism. It is considered of benefit to the elderly, because it may prevent the age-related decline of serotonin.

It helps relax blood vessels, improving circulation and the delivery of nutrients, oxygen, and glucose throughout the body, including the brain. It strengthens fragile capillaries and interferes with platelet-activating factor, a protein that can trigger spasms in the lungs. Concentrated ginkgo leaf increases the synthesis of dopamine, norepinephrine, and other neurotransmitters.

Ginkgo leaf can be used in the treatment of Alzheimer's disease, anxiety, dementia, depression, fatigue, memory loss, neuropathy, and pain in the extremities.

Contraindications

Side effects from using unstandardized ginkgo leaves are rare. However, large amounts or concentrations have been reported to cause gastrointestinal disturbance, irritability, restlessness, and headache. Ginkgo leaf can negatively affect the blood's ability to clot, so avoid ginkgo for at least a week before surgery, in cases of hemophilia, or when using anticoagulant drugs such as Coumadin, aspirin, or MAO inhibitors.

Fruit from the female trees may cause contact dermatitis or mouth lesions. Do not eat the pulp of the fruit. It smells awful, so you won't want to! Even standing over roasting seeds can cause eye irritation and dermatitis.

Avoid long-term use of the seed, and do not take more than ten seeds at a time. Excess use may cause fever, headache, irritation of the mucous membranes and skin, or emotional irritability.

10. Ginseng

Panax ginseng (Asian ginseng), *P. quinquefolium* (American ginseng)
Araliaceae (ginseng) family

Medicinal Uses

Asian ginseng has an incredibly long history of use in Chinese medicine, dating back some 6,000 years. It is valued especially for its restorative and energizing properties.

American ginseng has properties similar to those of Asian ginseng, but it is considered to be milder and it is more likely to be prescribed for younger people. Ginseng improves energy levels and enhances mental alertness.

Ginseng of either variety helps the body better utilize oxygen, spares glycogen utilization, increases cerebral circulation, helps the adrenal glands to better conserve their stores of vitamin C, aids in stabilizing blood sugar levels, helps balance hormone levels in men and women, reduces LDL ("bad" cholesterol) levels while elevating HDL ("good" cholesterol) levels, and aids in the production of DNA, RNA, interferon, and red and white blood cells. It helps the body adapt to stress and maintain normal blood pressure, glucose levels, and hormonal function.

It can improve stamina, reaction time, and concentration, which makes it useful for such pursuits as studying, taking tests, long-distance driving, and meditating. It also speeds recovery time from sickness, surgery, childbirth, athletic performance, and other stressors to the body.

Although the root is the primary medicinal component of the plant, the leaves of both varieties can be used to treat hangover and fever.

For best effect, take ginseng between meals rather than with food. It is best not to take ginseng at night, as it could impair sleep.

Contraindications

Avoid ginseng in cases of heat and inflammation, such as fever, flu, pneumonia, hypertension, or constipation. Do not give to children for prolonged periods, as it may cause early sexual maturation. Avoid during pregnancy and while nursing. Do not take ginseng in conjunction with cardiac glycosides except under the guidance of a qualified health care professional.

11. Goji

Lycium barbarum, *L. chinense*
Solanaceae (nightshade) family

Medicinal Uses

In Asia goji berry is traditionally used as a longevity tonic that nourishes the kidneys and liver. It stimulates the production of hormones, interferon, white blood cells, enzymes, and blood.

It also increases levels of the antioxidant superoxide dismutase and hemoglobin while decreasing levels of lipid peroxides, and it nourishes bone marrow and helps remove toxins from the blood by strengthening the kidneys and liver. Goji berries are used in Oriental medicine to help promote cheerfulness and a long life.

Goji berries are used to treat dizziness, erectile dysfunction, exhaustion, fatigue, hypoglycemia, low libido, low testosterone levels, senility, tinnitus, and vertigo.

Other Uses

Asian folklore claims that goji berries enhance beauty and cheerfulness when taken for long periods of time.

Contraindications

Avoid in cases of acute fever or dampness, such as diarrhea and bloating. Otherwise goji is considered very safe, even for daily consumption.

12. Gotu kola

Centella asiatica (formerly *Hydrocotyle asiatica*)
Apiaceae (parsley) family

Medicinal Uses

Gotu kola has been used in India as a cerebral and endocrine tonic. It helps to regulate serotonin and dopamine brain levels. It has a revitalizing effect on the brain cells and nerves.

In Asia gotu kola has long been considered a longevity tonic. An old Singhalese proverb says of gotu kola, "Two leaves a day will keep old age away." And there are reports of a Chinese herbalist, Li Ching Yun, who supposedly lived to be 256 years old and was a regular consumer of gotu kola.

Gotu kola strengthens the body's membranes, helps restore strength to the venous walls and connective tissue, calms the mind, improves neural transport, and helps the body detoxify.

Gotu kola is often taken as a brain tonic. On the first day of spring in Nepal, for example, gotu kola leaves are given to schoolchildren to improve their concentration and memory skills.

Contraindications

Large doses can cause headache, itching, stupor, and vertigo. Avoid during pregnancy, except under the guidance of a qualified health care practitioner. Do not take it if you have an overactive thyroid.

13. Hawthorn

Crataegus spp.

Rosaceae (rose) family

Medicinal Uses

Hawthorn strengthens the heart muscles, dilates the blood vessels, and improves circulation. It also calms the spirit and increases circulation to the brain.

As a flower essence, hawthorn promotes the healing power of hope, love, trust, and forgiveness. It helps relieve negative feelings from the heart and encourages knowledge of the strength and resiliency of the heart.

Contraindications

Using hawthorn may potentiate the effects of heart medications such as beta-blockers, digoxin, or Lanoxin. If you are using heart medication, consult with a qualified health care professional before commencing use of hawthorn.

Use hawthorn with caution in cases of poor digestion or acid stomach. Hawthorn's effects are slow to manifest; the herb may need to be taken for four to eight weeks before results are observed. It is considered extremely safe.

14. Hops

Humulus lupulus (syn. *H. americanus*)

Cannabaceae (hemp) family

Medicinal Uses

Hops clears heat and toxins, nourishes yin, restrains infection, aids digestion, calms the spirit, stabilizes the nerves, eases anxiety, and encourages sleep. Hops contains lupulin, which is considered a strong but safe, reliable sedative. It induces sleep and creates a pleasant numbing sensation. If you don't react well to valerian, hops can be a good substitute.

A hops pillow can be used to aid sleep. Fill a sachet, about 5 by 5 inches (13 by 13 cm) and sewn on three sides, with hops and tie tightly with a ribbon on the top. Insert it into a pillowcase. The calming aroma helps slumber. A pillow for children's sleep could be filled with dill seed, fennel seed, and lavender. Both King George II and Abraham Lincoln slept with hops pillows to aid sleep.

As a flower essence, hops helps stimulate both physical and spiritual progress and improves group interaction.

Contraindications

Avoid during pregnancy and in cases of depression. Use in conjunction with pharmaceutical sedatives only under the guidance of a qualified health care professional, because it may exacerbate their effects.

Fresh hops plants may cause contact dermatitis and allergic reactions in some individuals, and tiny hairs from the plant can irritate the eyes if they come in contact with them.

15. Kava Kava

Piper methysticum

Piperaceae (pepper) family

Medicinal Uses

Kava kava is an ancient Polynesian remedy for insomnia and nervousness. It is often used in the islands ceremoniously as a religious ritual, to welcome guests and honor births, marriages, and business deals. It helps foster open communication and a feeling of "letting go."

Kava kava helps warm the emotions, and small amounts can produce a pleasant, euphoric sensation. It is also used for divination and to produce inspiration. It calms the heart, spinal, and peripheral nerves and respiration, reduces blood clotting, relaxes the muscles without blocking nerve signals, and calms physical tension without numbing mental processes. Taking kava kava before bed can help induce pleasant sleep and vivid dreams.

Kava kava is also said to increase tolerance of pain. Aborigines often took kava kava before being tattooed, and women in labor sometimes drink kava kava juice for its calming qualities and to facilitate birth.

Kava kava can be used to ease anger, anxiety, mild depression, fear, nervousness, pain, and restlessness. It also takes the edge off withdrawal symptoms (from alcohol, nicotine, or tranquilizers).

Kava kava is fat soluble, so when preparing it as a tea, add coconut milk to the steeping solution to help the infusion assimilate kava kava's compounds.

Contraindications

Avoid during pregnancy and while nursing, and do not give to young children. Avoid in cases of Parkinson's disease and severe depression. Do not take in conjunction with alcohol, sedatives, tranquilizers, or antidepressants, as it can potentiate their effects.

Remain aware of kava kava's soporific effects; try to avoid driving, operating heavy machinery, or other activities that require fast reaction times after taking kava kava. On the plus side, kava kava, unlike many sedatives, is not habit forming. Daily use of kava shouldn't exceed three months, though occasional use on an ongoing basis is fine for those in good health.

Kava kava may cause the tongue, mouth, and other body parts to feel somewhat numb and rubbery temporarily; this is normal. However, excess amounts can cause disturbed vision, dilated pupils, and difficulty walking. Large doses taken for extended periods can have a cumulative effect on the liver, causing kawaism, a condition marked by a yellowish tinge to the skin, a scaly rash, apathy, anorexia, and bloodshot eyes.

In Europe there have been some reports of severe liver damage resulting from use of kava kava, prompting a number of nations to ban sales of it. The problem appears to be caused by a compound, called pipermethystine, that is found in the stem peelings and leaves of the kava plant but not in the roots.

Traditional kava preparations are extracted from the roots, and the peelings and leaves are discarded. However, some European pharmaceutical companies bought up the kava waste products when demand for kava extract soared in the early 2000s. The cases of liver damage appear to have involved people who took standardized extract capsules, which may have contained kava stem peelings and roots as well as chemical solvents. For this reason, avoid kava products made from the leaves or stems of the plant. The traditional tea prepared from the root appears to be quite safe.

16. Lavender

Lavandula spp., including *L. angustifolia* (syn. *L. officinalis, L. vera, L. spica*), *L. stoechas* (French lavender), *L. viridis*
Lamiaceae (mint) family

Medicinal Uses

The herb clears heat, calms nerves, and settles digestion. It can be used to treat anxiety, mild depression, fear, headache (tension or migraine), insomnia, irritability, nervousness, pain, restlessness, and stress. Simply inhaling the scent of lavender essential oil from the bottle helps prevent fainting and relieves stress and depression.

Today, lavender is popular as a spirit-lifting, nerve-relaxing, calming fragrance. It is popular in baths, sachets, potpourris, sleep pillows, soaps, perfumes, and other aromatic products. It is a helpful fragrance in a birthing room, as it can help calm the laboring woman. Lavender can also be used as a bath herb to soothe cranky children. Placing a drop of lavender essential oil on the edge of the mattress of a teething baby can help calm him or her.

Contraindications

Avoid large doses of lavender during pregnancy, as its effect on the developing fetus has not yet been determined.

17. Lemon Balm

Melissa officinalis
Lamiaceae (mint) family

Medicinal Uses

Lemon balm was widely used in ancient Greece and Rome. Avicenna, the great Arabic physician (980–1037), said that lemon balm caused "the mind and heart to be merry."

Lemon balm clears heat, calms the heart, improves concentration, cleanses the liver, improves chi circulation, lifts the spirits, and protects the cerebrum from excess stimuli. It eases anxiety and nervousness and helps with insomnia and fatigue. The essential oil can be inhaled several times daily to ease mild depression.

German studies indicate that lemon balm's volatile oils help protect the cerebrum from excess external stimuli. It affects the limbic system and helps balance emotional states. It makes an uplifting bath herb.

It is a good herb for children: A cup of tea before bed can help prevent nightmares and allow for a good night's sleep, and it is excellent to calm the nerves and boost the mood of schoolchildren who are anxious about upcoming tests.

Contraindications

Lemon balm is considered very safe and is a favorite herb for children. It can lower thyroid function, however, which is beneficial in some cases but not for those with a hypothyroid condition.

18. Licorice

Glycyrrhiza glabra (European licorice), *G. inflata, G. lepidota* (American licorice), *G. uralensis* (Chinese licorice)
Apiaceae (parsley) family

Medicinal Uses

Licorice is one of the most commonly used herbs in Traditional Chinese Medicine. It enters all twelve meridians and harmonizes the effects of other herbs, helping to prolong their effects. In Chinese Medicine, licorice root is known as "the great harmonizer" and is often added to herbal formulas. It induces a feeling of calmness, peace, and harmony; slows response to stress; and helps exhaustion due to stress.

Contraindications

Avoid licorice in cases of edema, nausea, vomiting, and rapid heartbeat. Licorice is not recommended during pregnancy or in combination with steroid or digoxin medications. Large doses may cause sodium retention and potassium depletion and may be emetic. Prolonged or excessive use may elevate blood pressure and cause headache and vertigo. Avoid continuous use in excess of six weeks, except under the guidance of a qualified health care practitioner.

Chinese licorice (*G. uralensis*) is said to be less likely to cause side effects than the European variety (*G. glabra*). All these precautions notwithstanding, licorice is often added in very small amounts to other herbal medicines, so if you are at risk, read the label.

19. Milk Thistle

Silybum marianum (formerly *Carduus marianus*)
Asteraeae (daisy) family

Medicinal Uses

Milk thistle seed has long been used medicinally. Milk thistle seed helps protect the liver, prevents toxins from penetrating the interior of liver cells, promotes the growth of healthy liver cells, and improves the liver's function. It offers excellent support for the liver for those who need to take pharmaceutical drugs.

Other Uses

In magical traditions, milk thistle is worn as protection against negative energy and used in purifying baths.

Contraindications

There have been occasional reports of the seeds causing bloating or diarrhea or having a laxative effect.

20. Motherwort

Leonurus cardiaca
Lamiaceae (mint) family

Medicinal Uses

Calms without causing drowsiness. Said to make mothers more joyful and balances tendencies to "overmother." Motherwort slows a rapid heartbeat, improves circulation, prevents blood platelet aggregation, regulates the menstrual cycle, and calms anxiety and stress that may contribute to heart problems. It is especially beneficial to women's health.

Contraindications

Avoid motherwort in cases of excessive menstrual bleeding. Avoid during pregnancy (but note that motherwort can be helpful during labor, under the guidance of a qualified health professional).

21. Nettle

Urtica dioica, U. urens
Urticaceae (nettle) family

Medicinal Uses

This is an herb that improves just about everything! My friend David Hoffmann, author of *The Holistic Herbal*, says, "When in doubt, use nettles."

Nettle improves the body's resistance to pollens, molds, and environmental pollutants. It stabilizes mast cell walls, which stops the cycle of mucous membrane hyperactivity, and it nourishes and tones the veins, improves veins' elasticity, reduces inflammation, and helps prevent blood clots.

It also helps curb the appetite, cleanses toxins from the body, and energizes, making it a motivating ally for those who seek to stay on a healthy diet. Drinking nettle tea before and after surgery helps build the blood, promotes healthy blood clotting, speeds recovery, and helps the patient reclaim his or her energy. Nettle is a highly nutritious herb that is particularly strengthening to the kidneys.

As a flower essence, nettle is recommended in times of anger or emotional coldness that can lead to spitefulness and even cruelty. It encourages fearlessness in people who feel isolated or have been "stung" by others, helping them regain the ability to connect with others by expressing their anger. It also helps users to release stress and reestablish harmony and unity within themselves.

Contraindications

All fifty species of the genus *Urtica* can be used medicinally, but stick with the urens and dioica species unless you have consulted with local herb authorities on the safety of local varieties.

Nettle is not known as stinging nettle for nothing; avoid touching or eating the fresh plant unless it is very young and/or you are very brave. Touching the fresh plant can cause a burning rash. Wearing gloves when collecting can help prevent this, but the hairs in large plants may still pierce through. A nettle sting can be soothed with a poultice of yellow dock or plantain.

Eating raw nettles can cause digestive disturbances, mouth and lip irritation, and urinary problems; however, these side effects are rare when the plant is puréed before ingestion and practically nonexistent when the plant is dried. When used appropriately, nettle is considered safe, even over an extended period of time, although those with overly cold, yin-deficient conditions should not use nettle for prolonged periods of time.

22. Oat

Avena fatua (wild oat), *A. sativa* (cultivated oat)
Poaceae (grass) family

Medicinal Uses

The alkaloids in oat nourish the limbic system and motor ganglia, increasing energy levels and a sense of well-being. With its high silicon content, oat helps nourish the skin, nails, teeth, bones, and hair. It builds the blood, relaxes the nerves, and strengthens the nervous system, making tactile sensations more pleasurable. It even supports treatment of addiction, alcoholism, anxiety, mild depression, exhaustion, insomnia, nervousness, and post-traumatic stress. When consumed regularly, oat can lower cholesterol levels.

As a flower essence, oat is helpful for those who are filled with uncertainty and dissatisfaction and are unable to find their life's direction.

Contraindications

Those with gluten allergies should use oat with caution.

23. Passionflower

Passiflora spp., including *P. edulis* (yellow passionflower), *P. incarnata*
Passifloraceae (passionflower) family

Medicinal Uses

Passionflower quiets the central nervous system and slows the breakdown of neurotransmitters serotonin and norepinephrine. It induces mild euphoria, quiets mental chatter, and promotes peaceful sleep. For chronic worriers and restless minds. It's safe even for children and the elderly. It is an herb of choice to relieve anger, anxiety, irritability, and stress. Passionflower was an official herb of the U.S. National Formulary from 1916 to 1936.

As a flower essence, passionflower helps integrate spirituality into daily life. It also helps clear emotional confusion and relieves pain and trauma.

Contraindications

Large doses may cause nausea and vomiting. Avoid large doses during pregnancy. Unripe fruits have some level of toxicity and should not be consumed.

24. Rosemary

Rosmarinus officinalis
Lamiaceae (mint) family

Medicinal Uses

Rosemary has a delightful aroma and a long European tradition of alleviating anxiety. Ancient Greek scholars wore laurels of rosemary when taking examinations to improve memory. This member of the mint family is said to stimulate the pineal gland, improve energy levels, and relieve stress. Rosemary also contains calcium, magnesium, phosphorus, iron, and potassium as well as more than a dozen antioxidants. Rosemary is a nervine, rejuvenative, stimulant, and tonic.

In the bath or footbath, it rejuvenates the body and mind and also helps relieve pain and sore muscles. As a flower essence, rosemary encourages users to be less forgetful and more aware, more present in their body, and more conscious. It strengthens the heart and mind and helps users receive strength from their loved ones.

Contraindications

Avoid therapeutic doses during pregnancy (though using rosemary moderately to season food is safe). Though rosemary is generally considered so safe that it is a common kitchen herb, extremely large doses could cause convulsions and death.

25. Saint-John's-Wort

Hypericum spp., including *H. perforatum*
Clusiaceae (Saint-John's-wort) family

Medicinal Uses

Saint-John's-wort has been used for more than 1,000 years to treat depression. It can be found in the official pharmacopoeias of the Czech Republic, Slovakia, Poland, Romania, and Russia. It's an antidepressant because it inhibits serotonin reuptake. It helps heal physically damaged nerves and benefits anxiety, mild to moderate depression, fear, irritability, and melancholy. It breaks up chi stagnation and calms and lifts the spirit. It also promotes tissue repair, deters infection, and helps relieve pain.

Saint-John's-wort's action results in part from its ability to block the reabsorption of serotonin. It might also enhance the body's receptivity to light. One component, hypericin, increases serotonin and melatonin metabolism. Another component, hyperforin, inhibits the uptake of dopamine, serotonin, noradrenaline, gamma-aminobutyric acid (GABA), and L-glutamate, thereby allowing these neurotransmitters to persist longer in the body, which contributes to emotional stability. It has been known to restore zest to the elderly who may feel lonely and uncared for.

Topically, Saint-John's-wort can be prepared as a compress to treat pain, and nerve pain. The oil or a liniment can be used for massaging the spine, neck, and head in cases of neurological damage, arthritis, neuralgia, and sciatica.

As a flower essence, Saint-John's-wort helps calm those who feel fearful or paranoid, making them feel more protected and trusting. It can help relieve nightmares and fear of death and brings feelings of courage.

Saint-John's-wort's effects are not instantaneous. Continued use is necessary, and as many as two to six weeks may be needed before the herb's effects manifest.

Contraindications

Saint-John's-wort should not be combined with antidepressant pharmaceuticals (for example, Celexa, Eldepryl, Marplan, Nardil, Parnate, Paxil, Prozac, or Zoloft), protease inhibitors, or organ antirejection drugs (such as cyclosporine), except under the guidance of a qualified health care practitioner. In fact, because Saint-John's-wort cleanses the liver, it is best to use it with caution in conjunction with any pharmaceutical drug.

Saint-John's-wort is not recommended during pregnancy, while nursing, or for children under the age of two. It may cause photosensitivity, especially in fair-skinned individuals. There have been rare reports of dizziness, nausea, fatigue, and dry mouth from its use. Some people may experience contact dermatitis from the plant. It should not be combined with MAO-inhibiting drugs.

26. Valerian

Valeriana spp., including *V. officinalis*
Valerianaceae (valerian) family

Medicinal Uses

Valerian calms the nerves and anxiety and eases panic. In fact, during World War I, valerian was used to treat shell shock and stress in civilians.

Valerian is sometimes referred to as a "daytime sedative" because it can improve performance, concentration, and memory during the day; help you sleep better during the night; and reduce the time needed to fall asleep. It calms nerves without dulling the mind. Topically, valerian can be used as a poultice to relieve pain.

Its effects are due to one of its constituents, valerenic acid, which has been shown to inhibit the action of the enzyme that breaks down GABA (gamma-aminobutyric acid), thus contributing to increased levels of calming GABA in the body.

In Europe today valerian is the most common nonprescription sedative, more likely to be recommended than Xanax or Valium. One reason is that valerian is not dangerous when combined with alcohol, whereas Valium (which isn't made from valerian) is.

Most people will find the smell or taste of valerian objectionable and will prefer using it in capsule or tincture form rather than as a tea. Valerian is best used for two- to three-week periods or when needed rather than on a daily basis. Large doses over long periods of time are not recommended for those with a tendency toward depression.

Some individuals find valerian works for them as a stimulant. This occurs because their bodies are unable to transform the essential oils in valerian into valerianic acid, one of the main calming components.

As a flower essence, valerian calms, encourages healthy sleep, and eases physical pain. It is helpful during convalescence. For those who did not receive adequate love during childhood, it lifts the spirits and fosters inner peace.

Note: Avoid boiling the root when making tea, which would diminish the plant's activity.

Many find the aroma of valerian unpleasant, much like that of dirty socks. Some find that making valerian tea with raisins added to the water improves the flavor.

Contraindications

Large doses of valerian can cause depression, nausea, headache, and lethargy. Some individuals, especially those who are already overheated, may find valerian stimulating rather than sedating. Do not use large doses for more than three weeks in a row. Avoid during pregnancy, except in very small doses. Do not give to children under the age of three. Avoid in cases of very low blood pressure or hypoglycemia; avoid long-term use in cases of depression.

Use with caution if you are going to be driving, operating heavy machinery, or undertaking other activities that require fast reaction times.

Valerian may potentiate the effects of benzodiazepine and barbiturates. Those taking sedatives, antidepressants, or antianxiety medications should use valerian only under the guidance of a qualified health care professional.

27. Wild Lettuce
Lactuca canadensis, L. serriola (prickly wild lettuce), *L. virosa* (bitter wild lettuce)
Asteraceae (daisy) family

Medicinal Uses
Wild lettuce calms the nervous system, aids sleep, relaxes the ganglions, and relieves pain.

The dried leaves can be smoked to ease pain and calm stress.

Topically, wild lettuce can be prepared as a wash or included in lotions to get rid of acne. The latex can be applied topically to get rid of warts or calm the itch of poison ivy.

Contraindications
Wild lettuce is best used only under the guidance of a qualified health care professional. Moderate doses can cause drowsiness, while large doses can give rise to excessive sexual urges or insomnia. Very large doses can be fatal.

The latex from the plant can cause eye irritation or contact dermatitis in some individuals.

28. Wood Betony
Stachys hyssopifolia, S. officinalis (formerly *Betonica officinalis;* syn. *S. betonica), S. palustris* (marsh betony), *S. sylvatica,*
Lamiaceae (mint) family

Medicinal Uses
The ancient Anglo-Saxons wore wood betony as protective charms. Wood betony breaks up chi stagnation, relaxes and strengthens the nerves, relieves pain, and promotes a more positive outlook. Wood betony can help with anxiety,

exhaustion, fear, headache, insomnia, night-mares, pain, palsy, stress, and persistent and unwanted thoughts.

As a flower essence, wood betony enhances pineal gland function, thus improving the user's sense of well-being. It fosters a desire for higher principles and inner calm and can be useful for those who are dealing with excessive sexual energy.

Contraindications

Wood betony is generally regarded as safe. However, large doses may cause vomiting. Pregnant women should avoid large doses, except during labor, and then only under the guidance of a qualified health care practitioner.

Do not confuse *Stachys* with another genus, *Pedicularis*, also known as betony, because their uses are not interchangeable.

AROMATHERAPY

Aromatherapy is the practice of using essential plant oils for healing body, mind, and spirit.

Note: Keep essential oils out of the reach of children and away from light, heat, plastics, and metals. Some oils can stain clothing and damage the finish on furniture.

Note: Essential oils that should be avoided during pregnancy include bitter almond, angelica, anise, basil, camphor, cinnamon, clary sage, clove, cypress, fennel, frankincense, geranium, hyssop, juniper, lovage, marjoram, myrrh, oregano, pennyroyal, rosemary, sage, sassafras, savory, thyme, and wintergreen.

Aromatherapy Inhaler

To make an aromatherapy nasal inhaler, add five drops essential oil (basil, lavender, rosemary, or eucalyptus are all excellent) to ¼ teaspoon Celtic sea salt. Place the ingredients in a small glass vial with a lid. Open and inhale as often as needed.

Bath: Add two to eight drops of essential oil to a hot bath after filling. Mix well before entering the tub so the oil doesn't stick to one part of your body. Essential oils can also be mixed into a carrier oil to disperse, then added to the bath. Should too much oil be added and the skin burns, wash off and apply vegetable oil directly to the skin.

Massage oil: Mix 1 ounce (1 teaspoon or 5 ml) of your favorite carrier with twelve drops total of birch, rosemary, juniper, or lavender oil. Or use twenty-five drops of essential oil in ½ cup (120 ml) of oil.

Room mister: To use these scents in your home, try putting twenty drops of essential oil into 1 tablespoon (15 ml) of brandy. Fill a mister with 8 ounces (1 cup or 235 ml) of water as a room spray or simply put a few drops of an essential oil in a humidifier, on a radiator, or in a pot of water on top of the stove.

Tissue: Place several drops of essential oil on a tissue and take deep inhalations.

Essential Oil Medicine Cabinet

Anise seeds (*Pimpinella anisum*) are members of the Apiaceae (parsley) family. As an essential oil, it promotes relaxation and sleep and curbs sugar and chocolate cravings.

Basil (*Ocimum basilicum*) is a member of the Lamiaceae (mint) family. Smelling essential oil of basil helps you gain a second wind when you are fatigued.

Bay (*Laurus nobilis*) is a member of the Lauraceae (laurel) family. Use bay to improve concentration and memory, and inspire confidence.

Bergamot (*Citrus bergamia*) is a member of the Rutaceae (citrus) family. The essential oil is inhaled to relieve anxiety, depression, and compulsive behavior, as well as to aid withdrawal from sugar, food, and alcohol addiction. It encourages the release of pent-up feelings.

Cardamom (*Elettaria cardamomum*) is a member of the Zingiberaceae (ginger) family. It is used to improve concentration, overthinking, and worry.

Cedarwood (*Cedrus atlantica*) is a member of the Pinaceae (pine) family. It helps promote strength during times of crisis, boosting confidence and willpower.

Chamomile (German) (*Matricaria recutita*) is a member of the Asteraceae (daisy) family. Its essential oil eases stress, depression, insomnia, and resentment. It is said to help one let go of fixed expectations and promote a sunnier disposition.

Cinnamon bark (*Cinnamomon cassia, C. zeylanicum*) is a member of the Lauraceae (laurel) family. The smell of cinnamon is pleasant, stimulates the senses, and yet calms the nerves.

Clary sage (*Salvia sclarea*) is a member of the Lamiaceae (mint) family. It arouses the emotions, eases depression, and helps you feel more grounded in the body. Clary sage helps relieve muscle tension and cramps as well as hormonally related concerns of premenstrual syndrome and menopause.

Cloves (*Eugenia aromatica*) are a member of the Myrtaceae (eucalyptus) family. It stimulates the thalamus in the brain to release encephalin, a neurochemical that promotes a sense of euphoria and also gives pain relief.

Coriander (*Coriandrum sativum*) is a member of the Apiaceae (parsley) family. Coriander is used in lotions and as a bath herb for sore muscles and joints. The essential oil is motivating, a gentle stimulant, and helps relieve depression and stress. It has long been used in love potions and as an aphrodisiac.

Cypress (*Cupressus semipervins*) is a member of the Cupressaceae (cypress) family. The essential oil is used for its sedative properties and helps suppressed feelings to surface and be liberated.

Eucalyptus (*Eucalyptus globulus*) is a member of the Myrataceae (eucalyptus) family. Eucalyptus can be inhaled as a decongestant, helping people to feel less constricted emotionally and to prevent fainting.

Fennel (*Foeniculum vulgare*) is a member of the Apiaceae (parsley) family. Smelling it naturally stabilizes blood sugar levels. It promotes confidence, self-expression, and creativity.

Frankincense (*Boswellia carterii*) is a member of the Burseraceae (frankincense) family. It aids in prayer, meditation, and spiritual self-discipline.

Geranium (*Geranium* and *Pelargonium species*) is a member of the Geraniaceae (geranium) family. The root and leaves are powerful astringents and anti-inflammatory agents. The essential oils are used to calm anxiety, lift depression, reduce stress and fatigue, and stimulate sensuality. Geranium helps you feel at ease, improves relationships, and aids in resolving passive-aggressive issues. Geranium helps calm anxiety and relieves nervous exhaustion due to overwork and stress.

Ginger (*Zingiber officinale*) is a Zingiberaceae (ginger) family member. Its stimulating fragrance helps open the heart and is aphrodisiac. It improves depression and promotes motivation.

Grapefruit (*Citrus paradisi*), a member of the Rutaceae (citrus) family. The essential oil helps to prevent overeating as a way to delay dealing with difficult emotions. Cleansing and clarifying, grapefruit helps clear feelings of frustration, anger, and self-blame, helping you be more realistic and feel lighter and satisfied.

Jasmine (*Jasminum species*) is a member of the Oleaceae (olive) family. Many consider the aroma of jasmine to foster feelings of love, confidence, compassion, receptivity, and physical and emotional well-being. The essential oil has a chemical structure similar to human sweat and helps stimulate dopamine production. It relieves stress, moves emotional blocks, calms fear and anxiety, and is mildly euphoric.

Juniper (*Juniperus communis*) is a member of the Cupressaceae (cypress) family. It helps you break through psychological stagnation and let go of worry and fear of failure.

Lavender (*Lavendula species*) is a member of the Lamiaceae (mint) family. It is an excellent bath herb that helps to lift the spirits after a difficult day. It helps release pent-up feelings and ease frustration and irritability. Lavender is of benefit to almost any condition and stimulates serotonin production. Calming and soothing, it helps relieve anxiety, fear, insomnia, and stress. Think of lavender as the "rescue remedy" of essential oils.

Lemon (*Citrus limon*) is a member of the Rutaceae (citrus) family. Lemon essential oil is antidepressant and emotionally cleansing. It helps relieve irritability and insomnia.

Lime (*Citrus aurantifolia*) has the same uses as lemon. It is uplifting and energizing, helping to dispel worry and clear emotional confusion.

Lemon balm/a.k.a. melissa (*Melissa officinalis*) is a member of the Lamiaceae (mint) family. The essential oil calms the spirit, nervous agitation, restlessness, and stress and eases insomnia. It promotes clarity.

Lemongrass (*Cymbopogon citratus*) is a member of the Poaceae (grass) family. The essential oil is also considered an antidepressant and helps promote mental alertness.

Marjoram (*Origanum marjorana*) is a member of the Lamiaceae (mint) family. It helps relieve obsessive thinking and obsessive behavior and promotes self-nurturing. It encourages a sense of peace and calms the feeling of neediness.

Myrrh (*Commiphora myrrha*) is a member of the Burseraceae (frankincense) family. Myrrh is used as an essential oil to help ease worry and mental distraction.

Neroli (*Citrus bigaradia, C. aurantium*) is a member of the Rutaceae (rue) family. Neroli oil, from orange blossoms, is sweet and cooling, relieves anxiety, stress, and grief, and is an antidepressant. Neroli promotes strength and comfort and helps you release repressed emotions.

Nutmeg (*Myristica fragrans*) is a member of the Myristacaceae (nutmeg) family. It invigorates the brain, calms and strengthens the nerves, and has long been considered an aphrodisiac.

Orange (*Citrus species*) is a member of the Rutaceae (citrus) family. Orange oil is anti-inflammatory and sedative. It eases tension and frustration, promoting more positive feelings.

Patchouli leaves (*Pogostemon patchouli, P. cablin*) is a member of the Lamiaceae (mint) family. Patchouli calms anxiety, lifts the spirits, stimulates the nervous system, improves clarity, and attracts sexual love.

Peppermint (*Mentha piperita*) is a very aromatic member of the Lamiaceae (mint) family. It is cooling and stimulating, awakening mental activity and relieving fatigue.

Petitgrain (*Citrus aurantium*), a member of the Rutaceae (citrus) family, is derived from orange leaves. It is sometimes referred to as "poor man's neroli." It calms panic and anxiety.

Pine (*Pinus species*) is a member of the Pinaceae (pine) family. It promotes confidence and feelings of positivity.

Rose (*Rosa gallica officinalis, R. damascena, R. centifolia*), is a member of the Rosaceae (rose) family. Rose is associated with physical and spiritual love and is a supreme heart opener. It helps heal grief from emotional trauma. Rose helps you feel happier and relieves anger, depression, jealousy, and relationship conflicts. Good for anyone who feels distanced from his or her emotional center.

Rosemary (*Rosmarinus officinalis*) is a member of the Lamiaceae (mint) family. Inhalations of essential oil of rosemary are used to improve memory and Alzheimer's disease, calm anxiety, promote confidence, and prevent fainting.

Sage (*Salvia officinalis*) is a member of the Lamiaceae (mint) family. The leaves and flowers are antibacterial, astringent, and antiseptic. The dried herb is burned as incense for purification of negative energy.

Sandalwood (*Santalum album*) is a member of the Santalaceae (sandalwood) family. Its essential oil is massaged into the forehead for its calming effects and to enhance meditation. The oil is used for inhalations to uplift depression and improve fatigue and coughs.

Sandalwood trees take at least twenty-five years to grow. For the essential oil to be made, the tree needs to be cut down, which is contributing to the decimation of sandalwood trees and the high cost of the oil. Either leave this herb alone or use only sustainably harvested products.

Spearmint (*Mentha spicata*) has a lower menthol content than peppermint and is thus less medicinal smelling and sweeter and lighter.

Tea tree (*Melaleuca alternifolia*) is a member of the Myrtaceae (eucalyptus) family. Tea tree oil stimulates the nerves and helps lift depression.

Thyme (*Thymus vulgaris*) is a member of the Lamiaceae (mint) family. Thyme is uplifting and invigorating.

Tuberose (*Polianthes tuberosa*) is a member of the Amaryllidaceae (amaryllis) family. Considered an antidepressant and aphrodisiac, tuberose strengthens and evokes the emotions.

Vanilla (*Vanilla planifolia*) is a member of the Orchidaceae (orchid) family. Vanilla calms and appeases anger and irritability. It is believed that the smell of vanilla may stimulate the release of the neurotransmitter serotonin, causing feelings of arousal and satisfaction.

Vetiver (*Vetiveria zizanoides*) is a member of the Poaceae (grass) family Its scent is uplifting yet calming to an overactive mind.

Ylang-ylang (*Cananga odorata*) is a member of the Annonaceae (custard apple) family. It has long been used to calm anger, anxiety, depression, fear, and frigidity and improve self-esteem and reduce stress. It also helps foster a state of peacefulness.

Wintergreen (*Gaultheria procumbens*) is a member of the Ericaceae (heath) family. The leaves and essential oil are both used for their analgesic, antiseptic, aromatic, astringent, and stimulant properties.

Essential Oils for Specific Conditions

Below essential oils are organized by ailment or condition.

Addiction: Anise, basil, cardamom, cinnamon, fennel, and rosemary.

Anger: Basil, cardamom, chamomile, coriander, frankincense, geranium, hyssop, jasmine, lavender, lemon balm, marjoram, neroli, patchouli, pine, rose, and ylang-ylang.

Anxiety: Basil, bergamot, cedarwood, chamomile, cypress, geranium, hyssop, jasmine, juniper, lavender, marjoram, melissa, myrrh, neroli, orange, petitgrain, rose, rosemary, sandalwood, thyme, and ylang-ylang.

Creativity: Clary sage, neroli, rose.

Depression: Basil, bergamot, cedarwood, clary sage, geranium, jasmine, lavender, lemon, lime, neroli, orange, peppermint, petitgrain, rose, rosemary, sandalwood, spruce, vetiver, and ylang-ylang.

Fatigue: Basil, cinnamon, clary sage, clove, eucalyptus, cypress, fennel, geranium, lemon, orange, peppermint, pine, rosemary.

Fear: Basil, bergamot, cedarwood, chamomile, coriander, cypress, clary sage, fennel, frankincense, geranium, hyssop, jasmine, lavender, lemon balm (melissa), lemongrass, neroli, orange, patchouli, rose, rosewood, sandalwood, thyme, vanilla, vetiver, and ylang-ylang.

Grief: Cedarwood, clary sage, cypress, frankincense, geranium, ginger, grapefruit, hyssop, lavender, lemon balm, jasmine, marjoram, melissa, neroli, orange, patchouli, rose, rosemary, sage, sandalwood, or ylang-ylang.

Insomnia: Bergamot, chamomile, cinnamon, clary sage, clove, frankincense, lavender, lemon, lemon balm, marjoram, myrrh, neroli, nutmeg, orange, petitgrain, rose, sandalwood, ylang-ylang.

Memory and intelligence: Basil, bay, eucalyptus, ginger, jasmine, lavender, lemon, lemongrass, lime, orange, peppermint, and rosemary.

Nightmares: Anise, fennel, marjoram, patchouli, peppermint, and rosemary.

Pain: Chamomile, eucalyptus, frankincense, geranium, ginger, lavender, peppermint, rosemary, and wintergreen.

Stress: Anise, basil, bay leaf, bergamot, cardamom, chamomile, clary sage, cypress, fennel, frankincense, geranium, ginger, jasmine, juniper, lavender, lemon, marjoram, melissa, neroli, nutmeg, orange, peppermint, pine, rose, sage, sandalwood, spearmint, thyme, and ylang-ylang.

Worry: Clary sage, jasmine, and ylang-ylang.

TEA FORMULAS

With just a small repertoire of herbs, you can create effective, safe, and delicious healing blends that nourish, cleanse, and support the body in a multitude of manners. There is also no reason why you can't boil some water, add a tea bag as well and one or more bulk teas, and allow them all to steep. It's perfectly safe to mix several teas together.

When making a tea that contains roots and leaves or flowers, simmer the roots covered first, then turn off the heat and add the remaining ingredients.

Addiction-Free Teas
The following herbs help reduce cravings for harmful substances.

Basil leaf
Catnip leaf
Cinnamon bark
Clove bud
Dandelion root (raw)
Fennel seed
Lemon balm herb
Oatstraw or seed
Orange peel
Spearmint leaf

Blood-Sugar-Stabilizing Teas
Help stabilize the highs and lows of blood glucose levels with these herbs.

Burdock root
Cinnamon bark
Dandelion root
Fennel seed
Fenugreek seed
Marshmallow root
Fresh blueberries

Brain Booster Teas
Sharpen your wits with classic smart herbs.

Oatstraw or seed
Nettle leaf
Rosemary
Ginkgo
Gotu kola
Sage
Yerba maté leaf

Calm Stress Teas
Sip a cup of soothing, stress-relieving tea.

Lemon balm leaf
Chamomile flower
Catnip leaf
Oatstraw or seed

Depression Uplift Teas

These herbs help raise your spirits when you feel blue.

Dandelion root
Oatstraw or seed
Lemon balm leaf
Nettle leaf
Spearmint leaf

Energy Teas

These herbs help you buzz around.

Green tea
Yerba maté leaf
Oatstraw or seed
Nettle leaf
Hawthorn leaf and flower
Licorice root

Get Grounded Teas

Get grounded with deep roots!

Burdock root
Dandelion root
Gingerroot

Headache-Free Teas

To help relieve the pain and inflammation of a throbbing head.

Chamomile flowers
Dandelion root
Rosemary leaf
Peppermint leaf
Lemon balm

Pain Relief Teas

The following herbs are analgesic, anti-inflammatory, and calming.

Clove bud
Chamomile flower
Linden flower
Marshmallow root
Peppermint leaf
Rosemary leaf

Recovery Teas (from surgery, illness, grief, trauma, and accidents)

Nutrient density, healing, and building are needed after a difficult life experience.

Dandelion root
Marshmallow root
Nettle leaf
Oatstraw or seed
Plantain leaf
Rose hips
Violet leaf

Bedtime Teas

Chamomile flower
Catnip
Lemon balm
Linden flower
Oatstraw or seed

RESOURCES

American Botanical Council
P.O. Box 14445
Austin, TX 78714-4345
800-373-705
www.herbalgram.org
Publishes Herbalgram; *sells herbal books.*

American Herbalists Guild
141 Nob Hill Road
Cheshire, CT 06410
203-272-6731
www.americanherbalistsguild.com
Offers a member directory of peer-reviewed herbal practitioners.

American Herb Association
P.O. Box 1673
Nevada, CA 95959
530-265-9552
www.ahaherb.com
Provides listing of herb schools throughout the country and an excellent newsletter.

International Society for Mental Health Online
ismho.org
ISMHO was formed to promote the understanding, use, and development of online communication, information, and technology for the international mental health community.

The Science and Art of Herbalism Correspondence Course
P.O. Box 420
East Barre, VT 05649
802-479-9825
www.sagemountain.com
An excellent home-study program designed by beloved herbalist Rosemary Gladstar.

Mental Health Resource
National Institute of Mental Health
Science Writing, Press, and Dissemination Branch
6001 Executive Boulevard, Room 6200, MSC 9663
Bethesda, MD 20892-9663
866-415-8051 (TTY toll-free)
www.nimh.nih.gov

United Plant Savers
P.O. Box 98
East Barre, VT 05649
802-479-9825
www.unitedplantsavers.org
Group that promotes awareness about rare and endangered species and offers a great newsletter.

World Federation for Mental Health
P.O. Box 807
Occoquan, VA 22125
www.wfmh.com
*International organization founded to advance,
among all peoples and nations, the prevention of
mental and emotional disorders, the proper treatment and care of those with such disorders, and
the promotion of mental health.*

Resources for Buying Herbs and Supplies

Asia Natural Products
590 Townsend Street
San Francisco, CA 94103
415-522-1668/800-355-3808
www.drkangformulas.com
Sells quality Oriental herbs.

Boiron Homeopathics
6 Campus Boulevard
Newtown Square, PA 19073-3267
800-264-7661
www.boironusa.com
Offers a complete line of homeopathic products.

Dr. Bronner's Magic Soap
P.O. Box 28
Escondido, CA 92033
877-786-3649
www.drbronner.com
*Excellent soaps for cleaning everything on the
body and in the home!*

Frontier Natural Products Co-Op
P.O. Box 299
Norway, IA 52318
800-669-3275
www.frontiercoop.com
Offers mail-order herbs and herbal products.

Herb Pharm
P.O. Box 116
Williams, OR 97544
541-846-6262
www.herb-pharm.com
Makers of excellent quality herbal tinctures.

Herbal Products
Allergy Research Group
2300 North Loop Road
Alameda, CA 94502
800-545-9960/510-263-2000
www.allergyresearchgroup.com
Sells homeopathic products for specific allergens.

Horizon Herbs
P.O. Box 69
Williams, OR 97544-0069
541-846-6704
www.horizonherbs.com
*Offers an excellent selection of herbal seeds and
seedlings.*

Mountain Rose Herbs
25472 Dilley Lane
Eugene, OR 97405
800-879-3337
www.mountainroseherbs.com
*Sells herbs and herbal products such as strainers,
empty tea bags, and tincture bottles.*

The Original Bach Flower Remedies
Los Angeles, CA
800-214-2850
www.bachflower.com
Distributors of Rescue Remedy and other Bach Flower Remedies.

Pharmaca Integrative Pharmacy
4940 Pearl East Circle, Suite 301
Boulder, CO 80301
303-442-2304
www.pharmaca.com
Sells quality supplements and herbal remedies through mail order.

Planetary Herbals
P.O. Box 1760
Soquel, CA 95073
800-606-6226/831-438-1700
www.planetaryherbals.com
Sells herbal remedies based on the work of Michael Tierra, C.A., N.D.

StarWest Botanicals
11253 Trade Center Drive
Rancho Cordova, CA 95742
800-800-4372
www.starwest-botanicals.com
Offers mail-order herbs and herbal products.

Appendix E

BIBLIOGRAPHY

Arbett, Lorenzo. *Kicking the Depression Habit.* New York: Prema Publishing, 1988.

Ayan, Jordan. *Aha! 10 Ways to Free Your Creative Spirit and Find Your Great Ideas.* New York: Random House, 1997.

Barrett, Susan. *It's All in Your Head: A Guide to Understanding your Brain and Boosting your Brain Power.* Minneapolis: Free Spirit Publishing, 1985.

Black, Dean, Ph.D. *Four Steps to an Alert and Active Mind.* Springville, UT: Tapestry Press, 1989.

Bloomfield, Harold H., M.D., *Healing Anxiety with Herbs: Featuring a Natural Self-Healing Program to Relieve Stress, Promote Sleep & Maximize Performance.* New York: HarperCollins, 1998.

Bragg, Paul, N.D., Ph.D., and Patricia Bragg, N.D., Ph.D. *Build Powerful Nerve Force: It Controls Your Life—Keep it Healthy.* Santa Barbara, CA: Health Science, 2007.

Brown, Richard P., M.D., Patricia L. Gerbarg, M.D., and Philip R. Muskin, M.D. *How to Use Herbs, Nutrients and Yoga in Mental Health Care.* New York: W.W. Norton and Company, 2009.

Butler, Gillian, Ph.D., and Tony Hope, M.D. *Managing Your Mind: The Mental Fitness Guide.* New York: Oxford University Press, 1995.

Challem, Jack. *The Food-Mood Solution: All-Natural Ways to Banish Anxiety, Depression, Anger, Stress, Overeating and Alcohol and Drug Problems—and Feel Good Again.* Hoboken, NJ: John Wiley and Sons, 2007.

Cousens, Gabriel, M.D., and Mark Mayell. *Depression-Free for Life: An All-Natural 5-Step Plan to Reclaim Your Zest for Living.* New York: Harper-Collins, 2000.

DeFelice, Karen. *Enzymes for Autism and Other Neurological Conditions.* Minneapolis: Thundersnow Interactive Publications, 2003.

Emery, Gary, Ph.D., and James Campbell, M.D. *Rapid Relief from Emotional Distress: A New Clinically Proven Method for Getting Over Depression and Other Emotional Problems without Prolonged or Expensive Therapy.* New York: Rawson Associates, 1986.

Germano, Carl, R.D., C.N.S., L.D.N, and William Cabot, M.D., F.A.A.O.S., F.A.A.D.E.P. *Nature's Pain Killers: Nutritional and Alternative Therapies for Chronic Pain Relief.* New York: Kensington Publishing, 2000.

Gladstar, Rosemary. *Herbs for Reducing Stress and Anxiety*. Pownal, VT: Storey Books, 1999.

Hickland, Catherine. *The 30-Day Heartbreak Cure: Getting Over Him and Back Out There One Month from Today*. New York: Simon and Schuster, 2009.

Hoffer, Abram, M.D., Ph.D., and Morton Walker, D.P.M. *Smart Nutrients: A Guide to Nutrients That Can Prevent and Reverse Senility*. Garden City Park, NY: Avery Publishing, 1994.

Hoffmann, David, B.Sc., M.N.I.M.H. *Successful Stress Control: The Natural Way*. Rochester, VT: Thorsons Publishers, 1987.

Hunt, Douglas, M.D. *No More Fears: From Crippling Phobias to the Jitters, Fight Your Fears with Nutrition!* New York: Warner Books, 1988.

Katz, Lawrence C., Ph.D., and Manning Rubin. *Keep Your Brain Alive: 83 Neurobic Exercises to Help Prevent Memory Loss and Increase Mental Fitness*. New York: Workman Publishing, 1999.

Kiew Kit, Wong. *The Complete Book of Chinese Medicine: A Holistic Approach to Physical, Emotional and Mental Health*. Kedah, Malaysia: Cosmos Internet Publishing, 2002.

Kircher, Tamara. *Herbs for the Soul: Emotional Healing with Chinese and Western Herb and Bach Flower Remedies*. London: Hammersmith, 2001.

Kirsta, Alix. *The Book of Stress Survival: Identifying and Reducing the Stress in Your Life*. New York: Simon and Schuster, 1986.

Larrc, Claude, and Elisabeth Rochat de la Vallée. *The Seven Emotions: Psychology and Health in Ancient China*. Cambridge, England: Monkey Press, 1996.

Larson, Joan Mathews, Ph.D. *7 Weeks to Emotional Healing: Proven Natural Formulas for Eliminating Depression, Anxiety, Fatigue, and Anger from Your Life*. New York: Ballantine Publishing Group, 1999.

Levine, Peter A. *Walking the Tiger: Healing Trauma*. Berkeley, CA: North Atlantic Books, 1997.

Mayell, Mark. *Natural Energy: A Consumer's Guide to Legal, Mind-Altering, and Mood-Brightening Herbs and Supplements*. New York: Three Rivers Press, 1998.

Medina, John, Ph.D. *Depression: How it Happens How it's Healed*. Hong Kong: New Harbinger Publications, Inc., 1998.

Murray, Michael T., N.D. *Natural Alternatives to Prozac*. New York: William Morrow and Company, 1996.

O'Bannon, Kathleen, C.N.C. *The Anger Cure: A Step-by-Step Program to Reduce Anger, Rage, Negativity, Violence and Depression in Your Life*. Laguna Beach, CA: Basic Health Publications, 2007.

Russo, Etan, M.D. *Handbook of Psychotropic Herbs: A Scientific Analysis of Herbal Remedies for Psychiatric Conditions*. Binghamton, NY: Haworth Press, 2001.

Sachs, Judith. *Nature's Prozac: Natural Therapies and Techniques to Rid Yourself of Anxiety, Depression, Panic Attacks and Stress*. Englewood Cliffs, NJ: Prentice Hall, 1997.

Schnyer, Rosa, and Bob Flaws. *Chinese Medicine Cures Depression*. Berkshire, England: Foulsham Publishing, 2000.

Simontacchi, Carol. *The Crazy Makers: How the Food Industry Is Destroying Our Brains and Harming Our Children*. New York: Jeremy Tharcher/Penguin, 2007.

Stone, Thomas A. *Cure by Crying: How to Cure Your Own Depression, Nervousness, Headaches, Violent Temper, Insomnia, Marital Problems, Addictions by Uncovering Your Repressed Memories*. Des Moines: Cure by Crying, Inc., 1995.

Wills-Brandon, Carla, Ph.D. *Natural Mental Health: How to Take Control of Your Own Emotional Well-Being*. Carlsbad, CA: Hay House, 2000.

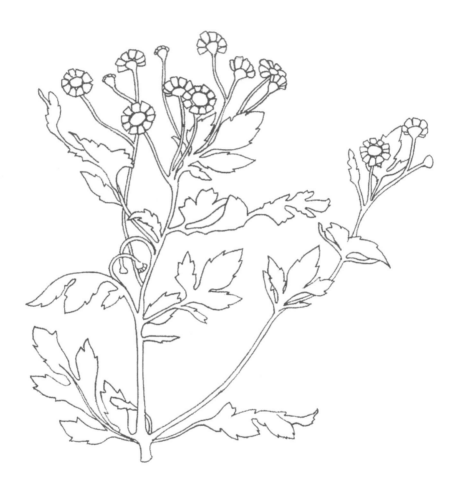

ACKNOWLEDGMENTS

Brigitte Mars: There are many to thank for the birthing of this book. Special gratitude goes to my coauthor Chrystle Fiedler, our agent, Marilyn Allen from the Allen O'Shea Literary Agency, and Jessica Haberman and Cara Connors from Fair Winds Press. Also much thanks to Briggs Wallis, always helpful and insightful. Loving thanks to Bethy Love Light, Matthew Becker, Marjy Berkman, Michael Shulgin, Charles Roberts, Red Elk, Roy Upton, Sunflower Mars, Mitch Stegall, Rainbeau Mars, and Michael Karlin. Blessings and thanks to Laura Collins, Donnie Curren, Martina Hoffmann, Kimba Arem, Dr. Rob Ivker, Ed Bauman, Mo and Jennifer Siegel, Laura Fox, Christine Martinez, Johnny Nash, the gang at Pharmaca Integrative Pharmacy, Tonics, Shine, and KGNU radio.

Chrystle: Many thanks to Brigitte Mars for being the best coauthor a writer could ask for! You are wise and wonderful and I've learned so much. Thank you to Marilyn Allen, my superstar agent and friend; editor Jess Haberman, for her enthusiasm and guidance; editor Kathy Dvorsky; illustrator Dayna Safferstein; and the production, sales, and marketing teams at Fair Winds Press.

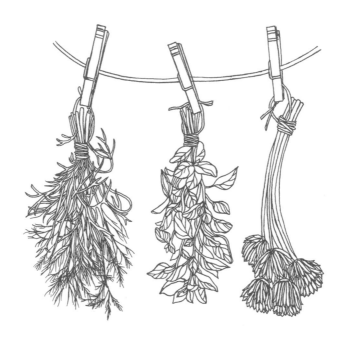

ABOUT THE AUTHORS

Brigitte Mars has been an herbalist and natural health consultant for more than forty years. She teaches herbal medicine at Naropa University, Bauman College of Holistic Nutrition, the School of Natural Medicine, Living Arts School, and Integrative Earth Medicine in Boulder, Colorado. She has taught at Omega Institute, Esalen, Kripalu, and the Mayo Clinic; she blogs for *The Huffington Post* and *Care2*. She is a professional member of the American Herbalist Guild and is known by many as an eternal flower child.

Brigitte is the author of many books and DVDs, including *The Country Almanac of Home Remedies, The Desktop Guide to Herbal Medicine, Beauty by Nature, Addiction Free Naturally, The Sexual Herbal, Healing Herbal Teas,* and *Rawsome!* and is the coauthor of *The HempNut Cookbook.* DVDs include *Sacred Psychoactives, Herbal Wizardry for Kids of All Ages,* and *Natural Remedies for Emotional Health.* Her latest project is a phone app called *IPlant*.

Brigitte and her daughter, Sunflower Sparkle Mars, run Herb Camp for Kids in Boulder. Brigitte's other daughter is world famous activist/yogini-actress/model Rainbeau Mars. Visit both www.brigittemars.com and www.rainbeaumars.com.

Chrystle Fiedler is the coauthor with Brigitte Mars of *The Country Almanac of Home Remedies* (Fair Winds Press, 2011), the author of *The Complete Idiot's Guide to Natural Remedies* (Alpha, 2009), coauthor of *Beat Sugar Addiction Now!* (Fair Winds Press, 2010), and *Beat Sugar Addiction Now! Cookbook* (Fair Winds Press, 2012).

Chrystle writes the Natural Remedies Mystery Series for Gallery Books/Simon & Schuster. Books include *Death Drops: A Natural Remedies Mystery* (2012), *Scent to Kill: A Natural Remedies Mystery* (2013), and the *Garden of Death: A Natural Remedies Mystery* (2015). To learn more about her fiction, visit www.chrystlefiedler.com.

Chrystle's magazine articles featuring natural remedies have appeared in many national publications including *Natural Health, Spirituality and Health, Vegetarian Times, Better Homes & Gardens,* and *Remedy* magazine. Visit www.chrystlecontent.com.

Chrystle lives on the East End of Long Island with her two dogs, Holmes and Wallander, and two cats, Tinker and Tuppence, all of which are named after fictional sleuths, three of which are rescues.

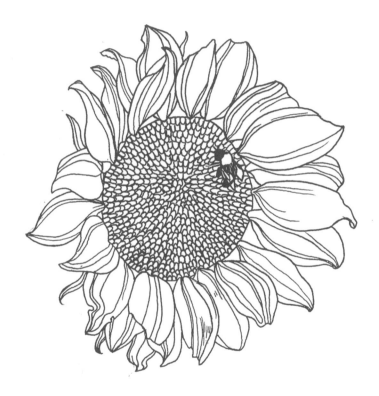

INDEX

galangal (*Alpinia galanga*), 88

garcinia (*Garcinia cambogia*), 109

gardening, to relieve stress, 36–37

garlic, 107, 116, 136–137, 139, 143, 170

Gelsemium (yellow jasmine), 32, 46, 64, 119

Gentian (flower remedy), 21, 64

geranium (essential oil), 30, 48, 65, 126, 154, 162, 172, 199, 202–203

germanium, 139, 142

ginger (essential oil), 30, 154, 199–200, 202–203

ginger (*Zingiber officinale*), 88, 109, 116, 148, 150, 162, 186

ginkgo biloba, 44, 62, 83, 124, 186–187

ginseng, 28, 44, 53, 124, 139, 187–188

glucosamine sulfate, 153

glutathione, 142

goji, 188

gold (*Aurum metallicum*), 31, 63

goldenseal, 140

Gorse (flower remedy), 21, 64

gotu kola, 82, 188

grapefruit (essential oil), 65, 112, 143, 162, 200, 202

Great Bupleurum Pills (Da Chai Hu Wan), 63

green tea, 80, 111, 124, 149

grief, relieving, 159–161, 205

GTF chromium (glucose tolerance factor), 112, 174

guar gum (*Cyamoposis tetragonoloba*), 109

gurmar (gymnema), 110

Hahnemann, Samuel, 22

happiness, cultivating, 177–181

hawthorn (herb), 28, 44–45, 161, 189, 205

Hawthorne (flower remedy), 162, 189

Headache, 158

Heather (flower remedy), 21, 53, 171

helichrysum (essential oil), 30, 162

hemp seed oil, 143

herbal remedies
about, 22, 182–197
for addiction recovery, 174
to boost brain power, 82–84
to boost immunity, 138–140
to defuse anger, 170
dosage guidelines for, 17
for grief/trauma, 161, 168
for healthy weight, 107–108, 116–117
to increase energy, 124
to reduce pain, 149–151
to relieve anxiety, 44–45, 53
to relieve stress, 28–30
for sleeping, 70–71, 74–76
to treat mild depression, 62–63

Hibiscus (flower remedy), 168

Hippocrates, 11

The Holistic Herbal (Hoffmann), 192

holistic therapies
to boost brain power, 89
for healthy weight, 112
to increase energy, 127
to reduce pain, 154
to relieve anxiety, 49
to relieve stress, 37–38
for trauma/addiction recovery, 168, 175
to treat mild depression, 65–66

Holly (flower remedy), 21, 171

homeopathic remedies
about, 22–23
to defuse anger, 171
for grief/trauma, 161–162, 168
for healthy weight, 119
to reduce pain, 148, 157
to relieve anxiety, 46–47, 53
to relieve stress, 31–34
to treat mild depression, 63–64

Honeysuckle (flower remedy), 21, 162

hoodia (*Hoodia gordonii*), 110

hops, 28, 45, 70, 117, 150, 161, 189

Hornbeam (flower remedy), 21, 64, 125

Hsiao Yao Wan (Bupleurum Sedative Pills), 63

huperzine, 83

Hypericum (Saint-John's-wort). *See* Saint-John's-wort (*Hypericum*)

hyssop (essential oil), 48, 162, 172, 202

Ignatia (St. Ignatius' bean), 32, 46, 64, 119, 162

immunity, improving
about, 129–134
aromatherapy for, 143
herbal remedies for, 138–140
nutrition for, 134–138
supplements for, 141–142
tips on, 144

Impatiens (flower remedy), 21, 171

inositol, 46, 85

insomnia, improving
about, 68–69
aromatherapy for, 71
establishing routines for, 73–74
exercise for, 72
herbal remedies for, 70–71, 205
nutrition for, 70
supplements for, 71

Interferon, 133

International Journal of Environmental Health Research, 50

ions, negative, 37, 50

iron, 86, 118

jasmine (essential oil), 30, 48, 53, 65, 89, 162, 172, 200, 202–203

journaling
for addiction recovery, 176
to cultivate joy, 181
to defuse anger, 173

3 1333 04421 0480